Top Performance in Business and Sports

The contents of this book were carefully researched. However, all information is supplied without liability. Neither the author nor the publisher will be liable for possible disadvantages or damages resulting from this book.

Please note: For reasons of readability this book is written in the male speech form. Any references to trainers and participants of course include men and women.

Prof. Dr. Elmar Wienecke

TOP PERFORMANCE IN BUSINESS AND SPORTS

MAXIMUM ENERGY FOR PROFESSIONALS AND ATHLETES
CASE REPORTS

Meyer & Meyer Sport

British Library Cataloguing in Publication Data

A catalogue record for this book is available from the British Library

Top Performance in Business and Sports

Maidenhead: Meyer & Meyer Sport (UK) Ltd., 2014

ISBN: 978-1-78255-055-6

All rights reserved, especially the right to copy and distribute, including the translation rights. No part of this work may be reproduced—including by photocopy, microfilm or any other means— processed, stored electronically, copied or distributed in any form whatsoever without the written permission of the publisher.

© 2014 by Meyer & Meyer Sport (UK) Ltd.

Aachen, Auckland, Beirut, Cairo, Cape Town, Dubai, Hägendorf, Hong Kong

Indianapolis, Manila, New Dehli, Singapore, Sydney, Tehran, Vienna

Member of the World Sport Publishers' Association (WSPA)

Total production: Print Consult GmbH, Munich, Germany

ISBN: 978-1-78255-055-6

E-Mail: info@m-m-sports.com

www.m-m-sports.com

CONTENTS

PREFACE **8**

1 INTRODUCTION **16**
1.1 Prescription for Energy:
 What Makes This Energy Formula So Unique? 16
1.2 Long-Term Research Results (Time Frame: 2000-2013) 18
1.3 Energy Status of 4,150 Executives and 6,120 Employees
 (Age Distribution: 44.3 ± 9.2) 21
1.4 Energy Status of 11,150 Top Competitive Athletes
 (Age Distribution: 24.3 ± 9.2) 30

**2 INTERNAL AND EXTERNAL ENERGY:
 LIVING A BALANCED LIFE** **42**
2.1 General Aspects of Our Energy Balance 42
2.2 Fit Instead of Exhausted: The Path to Increased Energy 45
2.3 Digression: The Complex Energy System 46
2.4 Physical and Mental Performance Capacity and the Role of
 Micronutrients in the Energy Metabolism 50
2.5 The Thyroid as Regulator
 of the Energy and Micronutrient Metabolism 53

**3 YOU ARE WHAT YOU EAT:
 ASPECTS OF NUTRITION PHYSIOLOGY** **62**
3.1 Functional Energy Metabolism Disorders Due to Micronutrient
 Deficiencies in Executives and Competitive Athletes 62
3.2 The Engine Cannot Run Without Fuel 64

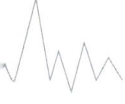

| 3.3 | The Components of Blood | 66 |
| 3.4 | Causes of Increasing Deficiencies in Executives, Top Competitive Athletes, and in Adults with ADHD | 72 |

4 BIOCHEMISTRY OF HAPPINESS … 80
4.1	Consequences of Biochemical Disorders	80
4.2	A Look at the Individual Measurements	84
4.3	The Role of Micronutrients: How Micronutrients Really Help	94

5 MORE ENERGY FOR A VITAL LIFE … 112
5.1	Exercise: Fit Instead of Exhausted, The Path to More Energy	112
5.2	Brain Food for Executives	124
5.3	Enjoying Life Without Being Stressed	139
5.4	Healthy and Sound Sleep	145

6 STRESS REDUCTION ON A BIOCHEMICAL LEVEL … 152
6.1	General Aspects of Cortisol	152
6.2	Sugar Related Stress	156
6.3	Prevention with Prescription for Energy	164
6.4	Competitive and Elite Sports with Prescription for Energy: The Proven Recipe for Training Continuity and Top Performance	169

7 ANALYSIS AND REGULATION … 176
7.1	Prescription for Energy: What is the Practical Application?	176
7.2	Case Studies of Executives	179
7.3	Case Studies of Top Competitive Athletes	190
7.4	Comments on Prescription for Energy	202

APPENDIX 204

1　Bibliographical References 204
2　Information on the Internet (Available by Download) 206
3　Acknowledgements 206
4　About SALUTO (Society for Sport and Health) 207
5　Self Checks: What is the State of my Energy Balance? 208
6　Photo Credits 218
7　PDF Download 218
8　Foundation for Micronutrients –
　　Prevention, Health, Quality of Life 220
9　Statements 223

PREFACE

Higher—faster—farther. This is the precept of today's performance society in business and sports. Team spirit, competition, winning, and losing: linguistically sport has already found its way into business.

Meanwhile, daily stressors increasingly lead to exhaustion and even the way to *burnout*. However, some scientists challenge the vogue expression *burnout*. Burnout literally means *being burned out*. The battery is dead on all levels. There is a prevailing sense of "I can't go on," "I feel weak, unmotivated, and unhappy." In 2000 only 70 in 1,000 employees in German businesses showed signs of exhaustion, but today that number has increased to 350 in 1,000 employees who are affected. Based on internal data, the burnout rate in executives is higher than 35%. Our own research findings from 10,270 entrepreneurs, executives, managers, and employees show that: 79% feel highly stressed, talk about increasing exhaustion, and have trouble unwinding after work. These are alarming symptoms. Recent research also shows that mothers, in particular, with the dual stresses of jobs and family, have a higher tendency of experiencing increasing exhaustion, extreme mood swings, and eventually to complete burnout.

In top athletes, too, the dream of winning the championship, the obsession with success as validation of personal strength, the financially lucrative offers, and the growing mental and physical demands increasingly lead to fatigue, severe performance, mood fluctuations, and often "inexplicable" injuries. These various stress-induced reactions and the associated disorders can be avoided with optimal energy intake. The brain reacts based on biochemical principles. When there is a lack of specific substances, certain functional sequences can no longer progress optimally, resulting in a premature state of exhaustion.

WHAT DIMINISHES OUR SENSE OF WELL-BEING

New research shows that one in two German citizens—regardless of age—complains of different disorders: chronic fatigue, frequent illnesses, trouble concentrating, lack of motivation, headaches, exhaustion.

"Humans don't get sick because the body lacks medicine, but because biochemical disturbances occur in the body that are not recognized and corrected!" (B. Kuklinski). A top athlete shows severe performance fluctuations and because of minor injuries is unable to ever tap his full performance potential.

The manager feels burned out, the woman with the stressors of job and family is overburdened, and the pensioner/retiree has many ailments. All too often, therapists are unable to adequately explain the causes. Here an optimal energy intake is verifiably helpful.

TODAY EVERYONE LEARNS AND BENEFITS FROM ELITE SPORTS

Every human being has an individual energy requirement. To identify the requirements and combat deficiencies using appropriate, simple measures has recently been one of our central objectives. Many international top athletes (Olympic, world, European, and national champions) have benefitted from these new findings and are thereby able to train at a higher level, free of injury and pain.

Overall we examined 11,150 top competitive athletes from all sports disciplines. But the most important finding is this: Today people from all areas of life and professional backgrounds (often with a variety of ailments) benefit from these findings that make it possible to preserve quality of life through an optimized energy balance. All of our parameters are archived in a one-of-a-kind database and support our analysis of individual energy requirements.

DEFYING DAILY STRESSORS WITH OPTIMAL ENERGY

Recently, we performed this integral analysis on a total of 4,150 entrepreneurs, executives, and managers and an additional 6,120 employees from various lines of work. There are interesting identifiable links between an individual's optimal energy intake and mental and physical performance capacity. By using specially-developed measuring procedures (functional analysis of the energy metabolism, special amino acids in the brain metabolism, and intracellular blood tests of the different micronutrients), we are able to ascertain and optimize the current individual energy requirement in a timely fashion, so that premature exhaustion can be prevented.

Small things make a big difference; simple can be great! Dive into a fascinating world of various energy flows!

Prof. Dr. Elmar Wienecke
(sports scientist)

OPTIMAL PRESCRIPTION FOR ENERGY– INDIVIDUALIZED AND SUCCESSFUL

Being healthy and productive with early detection and correction of biochemical disorders.

- Entrepreneur, age 57 (11,900 employees): After three years of use, I feel in great shape and more resilient that ever!
- HR manager, woman, age 48: I am a new person, I feel markedly better and am more even tempered.
- Vice world champion, European champion, winner of multiple German championships (in martial arts): If I had used this concept sooner, I would have been able to avoid many injuries.
- Italian soccer pro, age 22: Mentally and physically I haven't felt this good in a long time. This system is the way of the future!

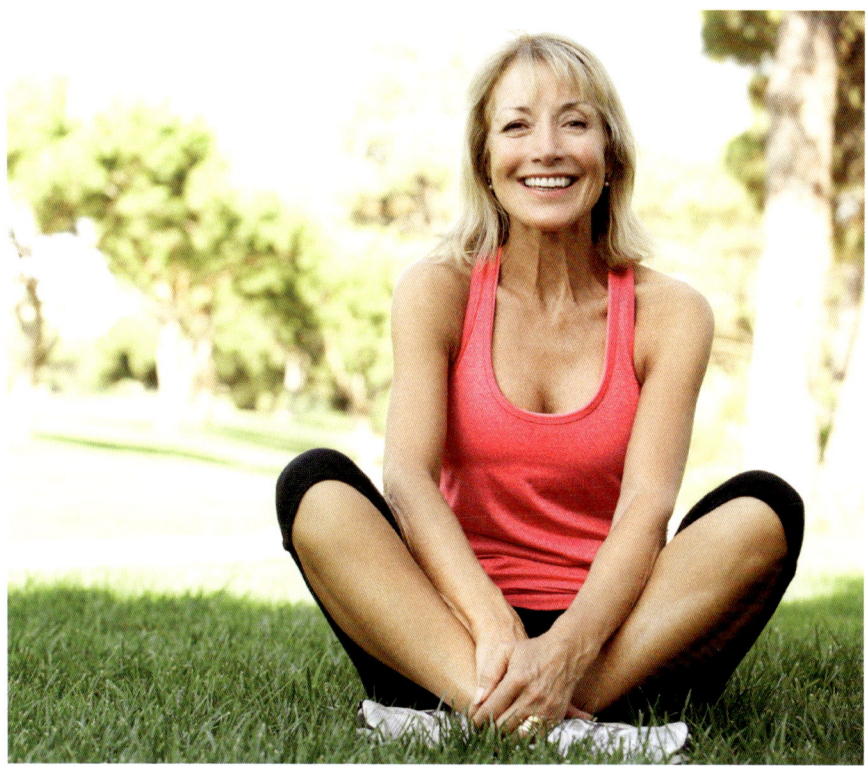

AN OPTIMAL ENERGY INTAKE BY EXECUTIVES LEADS TO:

- Improved mental capacity (better concentration)
- Increased stress tolerance
- Creativity
- Increased physical capacity
- Conservation of all important organ functions
- Optimization of complex metabolism of the brain, and endocrine and immune systems
- Verifiable job satisfaction

AN OPTIMAL ENERGY INTAKE BY TOP COMPETITIVE ATHLETES ENSURES:

- Training and competing at a higher level
- Improved regeneration ability
- Preservation of stressed structure function (ligaments, tendons, muscles, cartilage)
- Increased elasticity of many connective tissue structures
- Stable immune system
- Injury-free and pain-free training
- Training continuity
- Performance consistency

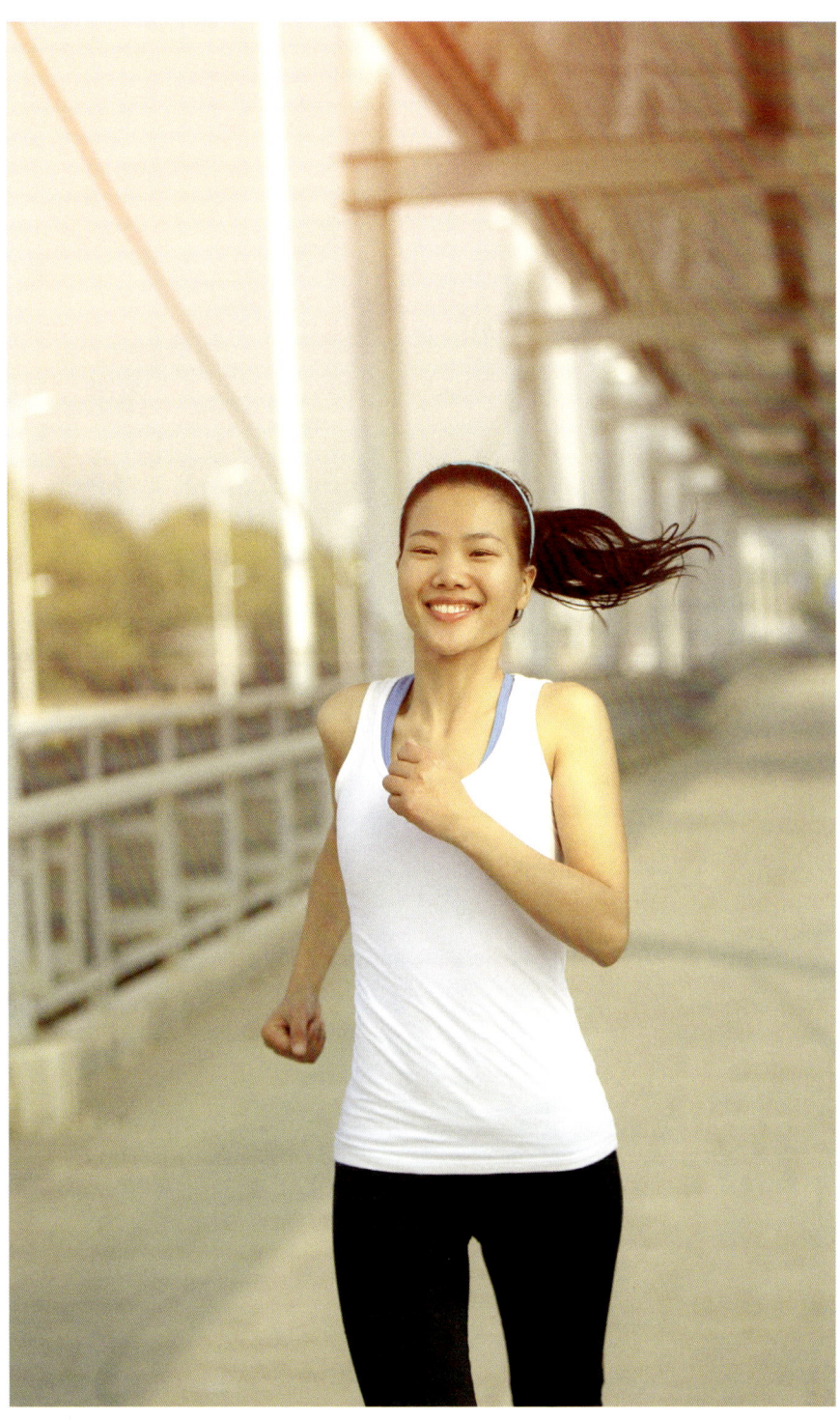

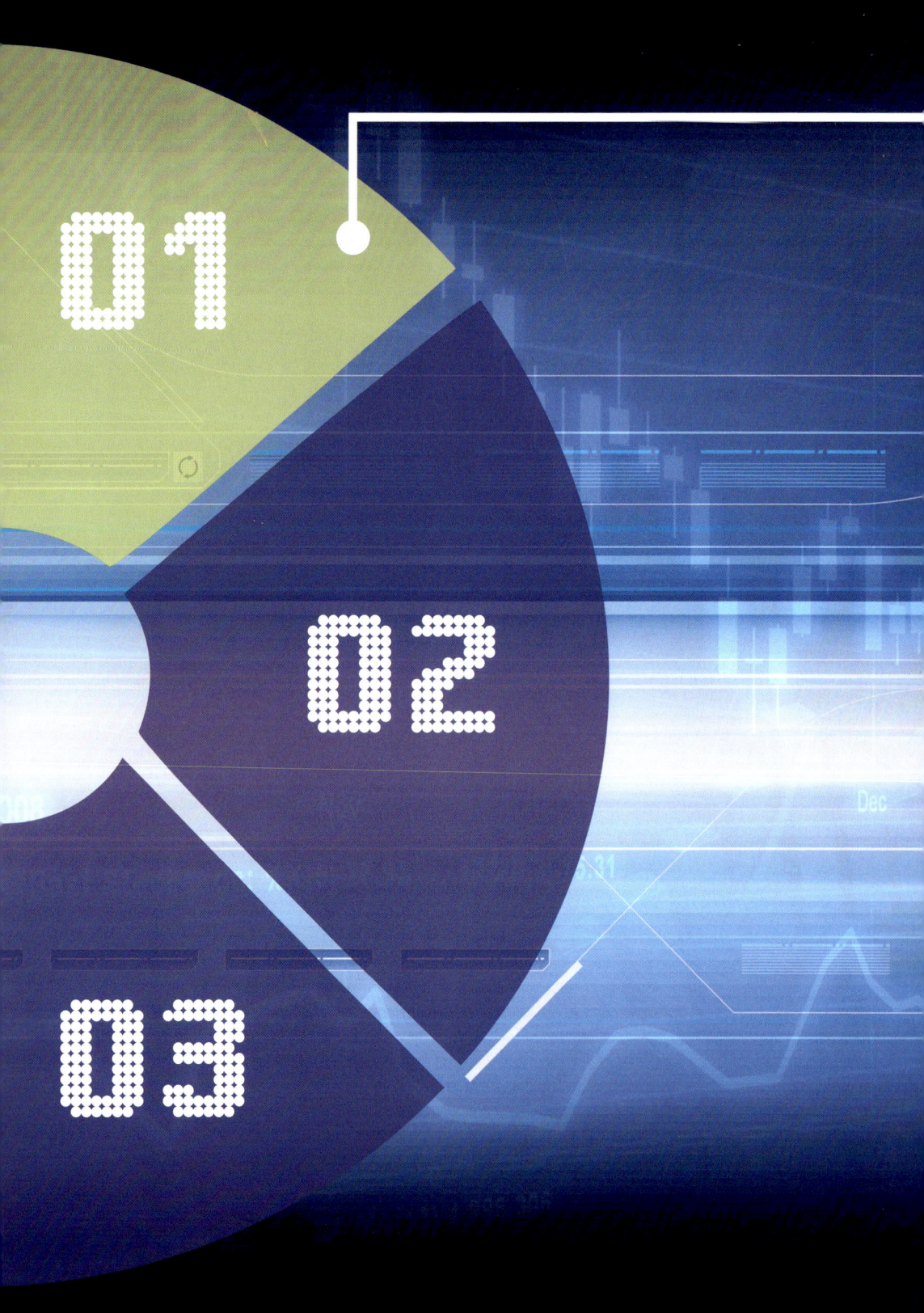

INTRODUCTION

1 INTRODUCTION

1.1 PRESCRIPTION FOR ENERGY: WHAT MAKES THIS ENERGY FORMULA SO UNIQUE?

Previous preventative concepts for the preservation of physical well-being and overall health are based on the hypothesis of a balance of biochemical processes in the body. The growing impact of stressors in the workplace and in competitive and elite sports increasingly upsets this balance. The subsequent stress reactions and the resulting disorders can be prevented with an optimal energy intake.

The brain's reactions are based on biochemical principles. When there is a lack of specific substances, certain functional sequences are disrupted, resulting in a state of premature exhaustion. One of our central objectives recently has been to identify these biochemical imbalances and to counteract them with appropriate measures. As a team (physicians, sports scientists, physical therapists, biochemists), we were able to develop a comprehensive analysis system, construct a database of currently 35,570 case reports, and create individualized formulas (Prescriptions for Energy) based on these results.

To begin with, measuring the functional energy metabolism of each individual is of fundamental importance. What is not working optimally? Is there, for instance, limited activity of certain enzymes in the energy metabolism? What do they look like? Next is a detailed analysis of the intracellular micronutrient concentrations. With top competitive athletes, there is an additional measuring of the body's use of its own structural proteins. But these extensive analyses do not yet yield specific recommendations for action. The evaluation, rating, and development of these analyses require long-term comprehensive data collection.

Our results show that a balance of the biochemical equilibrium can be found 25% above the respective median values of individual groups of people. The executives (entrepreneurs, executive managers, managers), and also the top competitive athletes, initially show biochemical disturbances with a number of disorders that are causally linked to a lack of energy and micronutrient intake (-20% deviation from median values).

With Prescription for Energy, the individual gets exactly what he needs, and after a few weeks and months of monitoring, we can see how the initial results clearly shift upward and performance capacity and quality of life verifiably improve. When we look at the entire spectrum of case reports, it becomes evident how highly (100% compliance) this longtime proven concept for success has been and will be rated with different groups of people in the future. Performance capacity, creativity in executives, and athletic success in top competitive athletes are no coincidence.

PROMISING OUTLOOKS

We are not at the end of the road! The road is the destination! New and innovative advancements show the transfer into diverse new areas of application. Detecting biochemical disorders via special analyses and correcting them with a targeted, individualized formula has, for instance, also led to very positive changes in children and adults with ADHD (Attention Deficit Hyperactivity Disorder). "Prescription for Energy" can verifiably increase the elasticity of stressed connective tissue structures in athletes, has a preventative effect, and, in the future, will be a significant factor in rehabilitation.

1.2 LONG-TERM RESEARCH RESULTS (TIME FRAME: 2000-2013)

We did an integral analysis of the energy status of 10,270 entrepreneurs, executives, managers, and employees and 11,150 top competitive athletes while simultaneously recording the numerous disorders of these individuals. We provide a detailed account of these integral analyses and their significance see in chapters 1.3 and 1.4. The evidence gathered from our testing and interviewing 4,150 executives and 6,120 employees shows blatant deficiencies within the diverse energy system.

SALUTO findings:

In 4,150 executives (entrepreneurs, executive managers, and executive staff) and 6,120 employees: (time frame: 2000-2013)

79% complain of increasing exhaustion.

31% subjectively use the common expression "burnout."

70% are dissatisfied with their diet.

70% of those interviewed are unable to relax after work.

More than **38%** exercise less than 3 hours per week.

78% feel severely stressed.

61% engage in goal-driven recreational sports (marathons, etc.).

Of those, **75%** have subjective complaints of increasing fatigue.

Prescription for Energy has **100%** compliance (improved mental and physical capacity).

Fig. 1

When we compare our own research findings with those of other institutes, we can see dramatic developments in recent years. (See Fig. 2).

The increase of psychological factors in disorders is particularly conspicuous and shows a direct link to serious shortcomings of the complex energy system. With special blood and urine analyses, we are now able to prove that a link exists between the different energy metabolism parameters, the measured deficiencies, and the individual well-

INTRODUCTION

being of these people. If the individual energy requirement can be ascertained early enough, it can be optimized so that premature exhaustion can verifiably be prevented or significantly mitigated.

Most recent studies:

Job-related demands are increasing.

Chronic fatigue syndrome (burnout) becomes dramatically worse.

Among German executives the annual burnout rate lies at 35%.

Chronic fatigue syndrome among employees is on the rise.

Statisticians list:

In 2000 = 70 sick days per year in 1000 employees
In 2011 = 370 sick days per year in 1000 employees

Fig. 2

PROVOCATIVE THEORIES

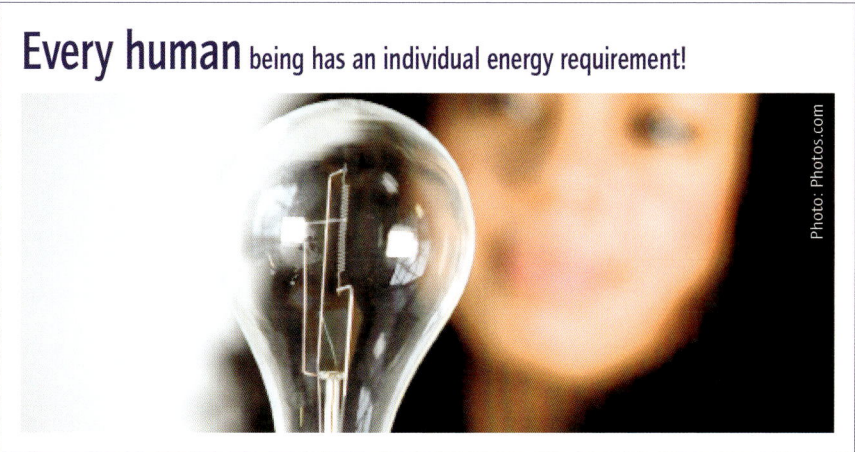

Fig. 3

We will offer a more detailed discussion of the following theories in the case reports (see chapter 7.2, pg. 179 and chapter 7.3, pg. 193) by referring to specific to case studies.

In executives an optimal energy intake results in:

- Improved mental capacity (improved concentration)
- Improved stress tolerance
- Increased creativity
- Increased physical capacity
- Preservation of critical organ function
- Optimization of the complex metabolisms of the brain and, endocrine and immune systems
- Higher work efficiency due to overall well-being
- Higher savings potential because of fewer sick days
- Verifiable job satisfaction

In top competitive athletes an optimal energy intake ensures:

- Training and competing at a higher level
- Improved regeneration
- Preservation of stressed structure function (ligaments, tendons, muscles, cartilage)
- Increased elasticity of connective tissue structures
- Stable immune system
- Pain-free and injury-free training
- Training continuity
- Consistent performance (little fluctuation)

In the past, a variety of athletic motor skills tests made it possible to verify results in athletes. Today, Olympic, world, European, and national champions from around the world benefit from these findings.

1.3 ENERGY STATUS OF 4,150 EXECUTIVES AND 6,120 EMPLOYEES (AGE DISTRIBUTION: 44.3 ± 9.2)

Between 2000 and 2013, we conducted an integral analysis of the energy status of 4,150 entrepreneurs, executives, and executive staff. Of these, 79% report increasing exhaustion, 39% report beginning signs of burnout, 70% are unable to unwind after work, 70% are dissatisfied with their diet, 61% engage in performance-based sports to compensate, whereby 75% in this group report increasing exhaustion. These days nearly all executives exercise: 38% work out approximately three hours per week; 100% in this group report a direct positive link between optimal Prescription for Energy and personal well-being.

We first create a starting basis of the complex energy metabolism of this group of people in an overall layout with the aid of specially-developed blood and urine analyses.

- The functional energy metabolism (pg. 85) shows existing impairment in the activity of certain enzymes (metabolism catalysts), resulting in insufficient energy production and consquently increasing fatigue.
- Measurements of the amino acids show severe deficiencies that block optimal serotonin production in the brain metabolism, which can have a considerable long-term negative effect on the individual person's mood.
- In this group of people, the intracellular micronutrient analysis (see pg. 67) shows severe deficiencies that causally result in the restricted activity of the functional energy metabolism. In physically very active people, a shortage in the energy metabolism results in an increased demand on the body's own structural proteins (see pg. 92), which can impede the preservation of stressed connective tissue function (tendons, ligaments, muscles, cartilage) and considerably increase the risk of injury in this group of people.

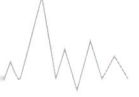
TOP PERFORMANCE IN BUSINESS AND SPORTS

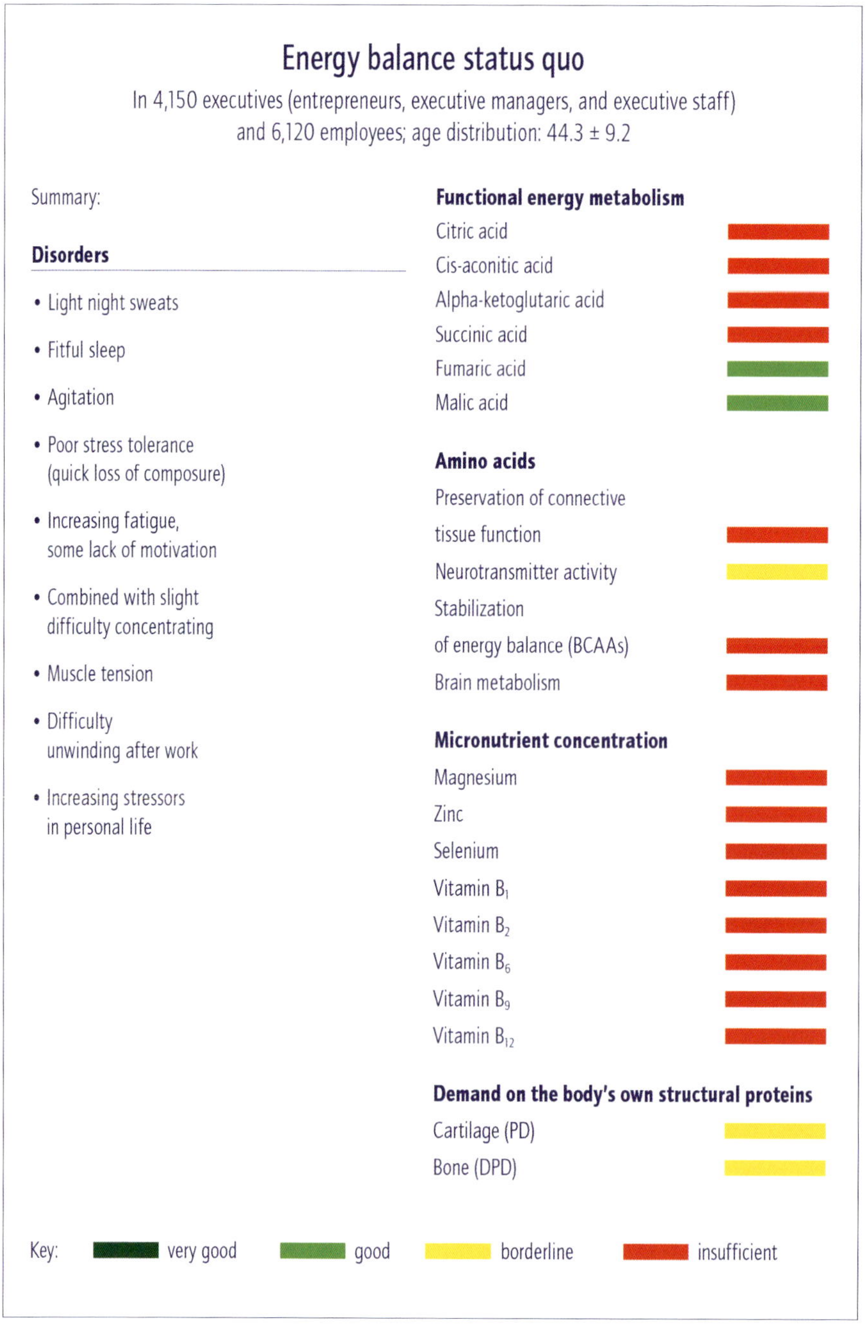

Energy balance status quo

In 4,150 executives (entrepreneurs, executive managers, and executive staff) and 6,120 employees; age distribution: 44.3 ± 9.2

Summary:

Disorders

- Light night sweats
- Fitful sleep
- Agitation
- Poor stress tolerance (quick loss of composure)
- Increasing fatigue, some lack of motivation
- Combined with slight difficulty concentrating
- Muscle tension
- Difficulty unwinding after work
- Increasing stressors in personal life

Functional energy metabolism

Citric acid	insufficient
Cis-aconitic acid	insufficient
Alpha-ketoglutaric acid	insufficient
Succinic acid	insufficient
Fumaric acid	good
Malic acid	good

Amino acids

Preservation of connective tissue function	insufficient
Neurotransmitter activity	borderline
Stabilization of energy balance (BCAAs)	insufficient
Brain metabolism	insufficient

Micronutrient concentration

Magnesium	insufficient
Zinc	insufficient
Selenium	insufficient
Vitamin B_1	insufficient
Vitamin B_2	insufficient
Vitamin B_6	insufficient
Vitamin B_9	insufficient
Vitamin B_{12}	insufficient

Demand on the body's own structural proteins

Cartilage (PD)	borderline
Bone (DPD)	borderline

Key: very good | good | borderline | insufficient

Fig. 4

INTRODUCTION

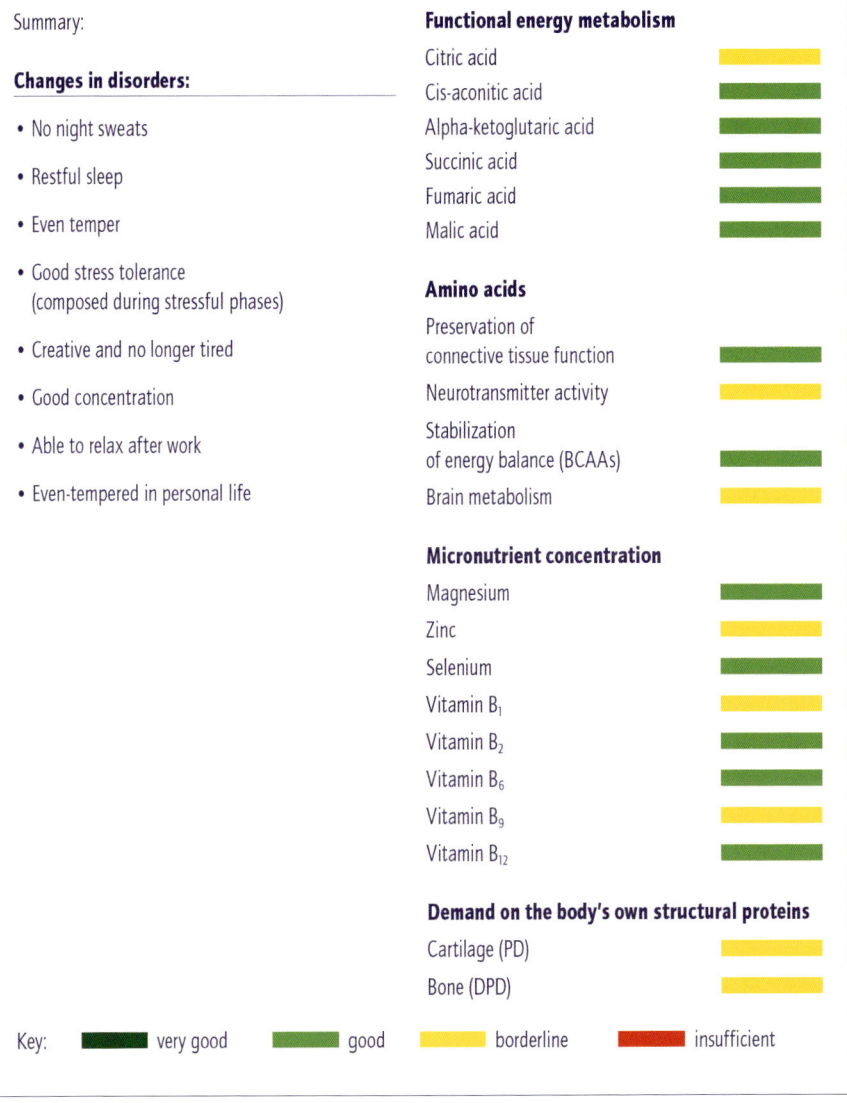

Fig. 5

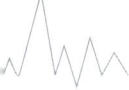

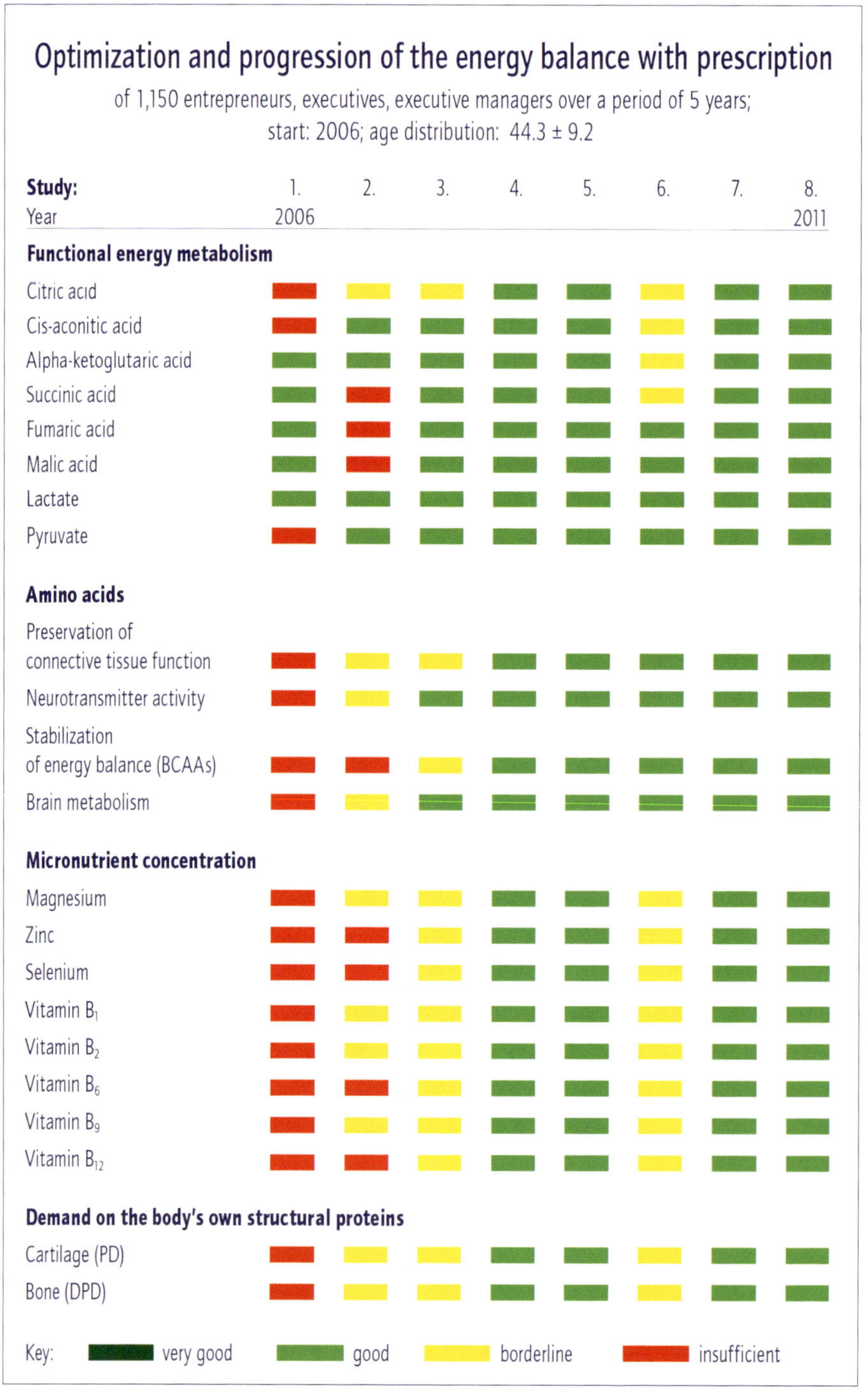

Optimization and progression of the energy balance with prescription

of 1,150 entrepreneurs, executives, executive managers over a period of 5 years;
start: 2006; age distribution: 44.3 ± 9.2

Study:	1.	2.	3.	4.	5.	6.	7.	8.
Year	2006							2011

Functional energy metabolism
- Citric acid
- Cis-aconitic acid
- Alpha-ketoglutaric acid
- Succinic acid
- Fumaric acid
- Malic acid
- Lactate
- Pyruvate

Amino acids
- Preservation of connective tissue function
- Neurotransmitter activity
- Stabilization of energy balance (BCAAs)
- Brain metabolism

Micronutrient concentration
- Magnesium
- Zinc
- Selenium
- Vitamin B_1
- Vitamin B_2
- Vitamin B_6
- Vitamin B_9
- Vitamin B_{12}

Demand on the body's own structural proteins
- Cartilage (PD)
- Bone (DPD)

Key: ▬ very good   ▬ good   ▬ borderline   ▬ insufficient

Fig. 6

The large number of biochemical disorders we initially ascertained in the 4,150 executives (entrepreneurs, executives, and executive staff) and 6,120 employees (see Fig. 4) is clearly reduced after only three months with an individualized formula for optimal Energy, though there is further potential for improvements (see Fig. 5). The positive changes show clear links between the optimal energy balance and well-being of this group of people.

The optimization and progression of the energy balance over a period of six years (2006-2011) in 1,150 entrepreneurs, executives, executive staff, with an optimal prescription energy intake (Fig. 6) shows how the initial deficiencies normalize over the subsequent years. The differentiated measurements of the energy metabolism are done twice a year along with the appropriate adjustment to the individualized formula. The different components of that formula can be seen in the case studies (see chapters 7.2 and 7.3).

LONG-TERM SUCCESSES

When the executives (entrepreneurs, executive managers, and executive staff) were given their individual formula, they were initially very skeptical. With respect to the aforementioned disorders, the individualized prescription energy intake was able to post fantastic successes within a short period of time. Detecting (via special analysis) and correcting biochemical disorders has had the desired results in almost every case. We also refer to this as *biochemistry of happiness*.

Here is the self-report from 1,150 entrepreneurs, executives, and executive staff after a prescription energy/micronutrient intake over a period of six years:

"In the beginning we were very skeptical, but after only 6 weeks we already noticed:

- No more night sweats
- Considerably improved sleep pattern
- Improved stress tolerance (improved composure during stressful phases)
- Clearly improved mood
- Improved mental and physical ability to cope with stress
- Verifiably improved immune system and fewer illnesses
- Subjective sense of improved mental and physical performance capacity

To us, Prescription for Energy is the ultimate! There is verifiably no better system that guarantees long-term well-being and creativity over a six-year period with an actual increase in daily stressors."

RESULTS FROM INDIVIDUAL ANALYSES AND THEIR PROGRESSION
VIA PRESCRIPTION FOR OPTIMAL ENERGY
OF 1,150 ENTREPRENEURS, EXECUTIVES, AND EXECUTIVE STAFF

Functional energy metabolism

A brief digression on the functional energy metabolism: The citric acid cycle forms the central switch point for the overal metabolism. The breakdown processes of carbohydrates, fats, and proteins take place here. A deficiency in basic micronutrients (amino acids, vitamins, minerals, trace elements) results in a defect in the power stations of the cells (mitochondrial dysfunction). Different metabolic products are measured here. An increase or decrease in the measured substances indicate certain disorders in the energy metabolism and is associated with decreased function during energy production.

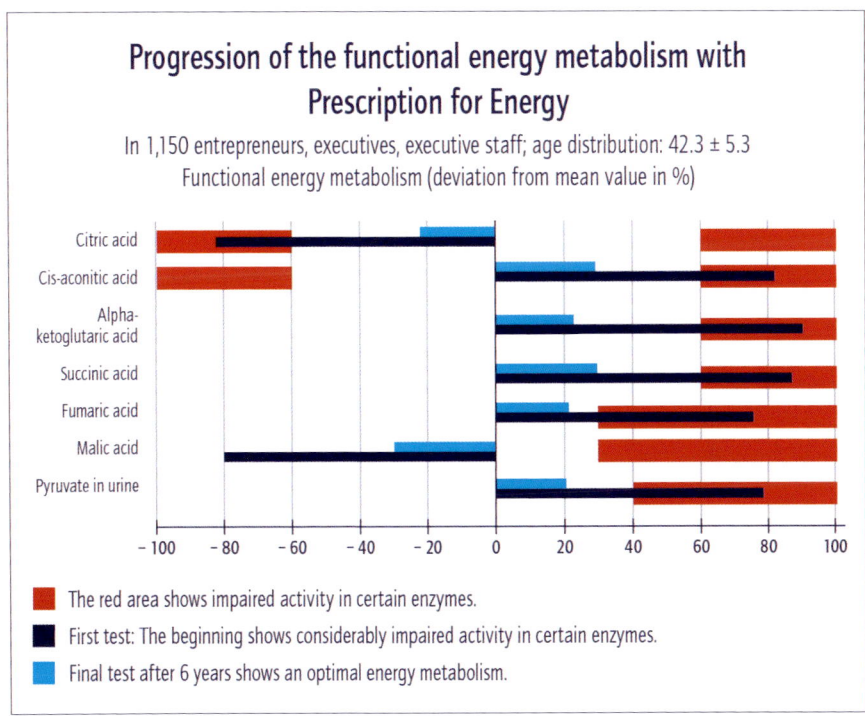

Fig. 7

Our findings show the deviations from the mean values (in %) in comparable people of similar age (personal life style, prior illnesses, athletic activity). Where the dark blue bar meets the red bar (see Fig. 7), we can see impairments in the activity of certain enzymes (these accelerate chemical processes) that result in a verifiable decrease in energy production. A normalization or economization of the metabolism can verifiably be achieved with an individualized prescription energy intake and is verifiably detectable after a period of five years.

Amino acids

Increasing exhaustion, bad mood, and irregular sleep patterns are often the result of biochemical disorders due to existing deficiencies in basic amino acids (tryptophan, phenylalanine, tyrosine), a targeted intake of which verifiably activates the brain metabolism so that combined with other micronutrients, these disorders can be eliminated in a short period of time (see Fig. 8).

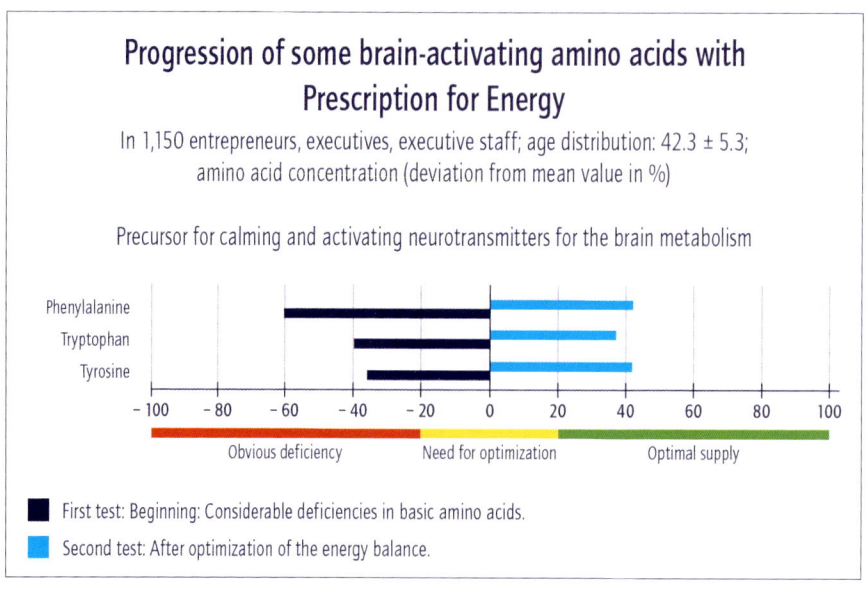

Fig. 8

Intracellular micronutrient concentrations

Important biochemical mechanisms of elements take place primarily on the cellular level. Determining the concentration of the element from the serum can thus not give any information about cellular processes (see pg. 68 and 69). With a targeted intake of individualized Prescription for Energy micronutrient concentrations can be optimized within one year to the point that the listed biochemical disorders in the metabolism normalize.

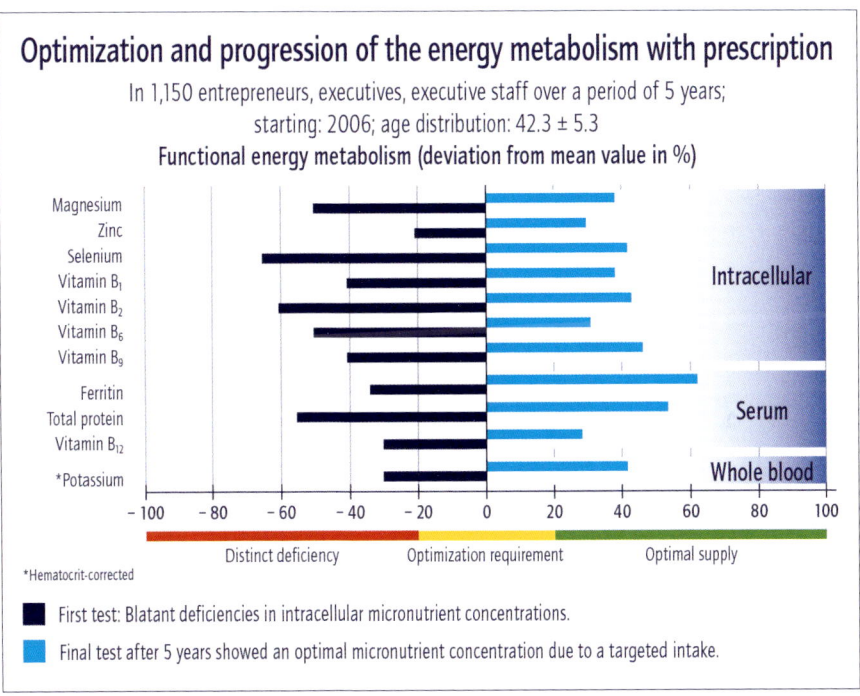

Fig. 9

1.4 ENERGY STATUS OF 11,150 TOP COMPETITIVE ATHLETES (AGE DISTRIBUTION: 24.3 ± 9.2)

In top athletes, growing mental and physical demands also increasingly result in fatigue, severe performance fluctuations, mood fluctuations, and sometimes inexplicable injuries (see Fig. 10).

SALUTO results:
In 11,150 top competitive athletes
(time frame: 2000-2012)

71% have injuries without external influence: 6-8 weeks of missed training per year.

70% report performance fluctuations.

100% report a direct link between Prescription for Energy and athletic success.

41% have an underactive thyroid.

69% lack mental alertness. They feel burned out.

59% report poor sleep patterns.

82% eat according to government guidelines.

Fig. 10

Between 1994 and 2013, we did an integral analysis of the energy status of 11,150 top competitive athletes.

- 71% were injured without external influence (e.g., tackling).
- Increasing chronic fatigue syndrome in athletes resulted in many overload reactions in the tendon-muscle-ligament apparatus, sometimes resulting in to fatigue fractures.
- 70% report major performance fluctuations.
- 52% are unable to train continuously because of frequent infections.

- 59% have trouble sleeping.
- 62% suffered from an underactive thyroid with corresponding disorders.

Anthropometric data from 11,150 competitive athletes between 1994 and 2013

	Age (years)	Height (cm)	Weight (kg)	BMI kg/m² (body mass index)
Total (N = 11,150)	26.3 ± 9.9	180 ± 4.5	71.45 ± 4.4	22.1
Female (N = 5,741)	24.3 ± 7.3	175 ± 4.3	68.1 ± 4.2	22.3
Male (N = 5,409)	28.2 ± 8.3	185 ± 4.8	74.8 ± 46	21.9

Fig. 11

Sport distribution

Soccer	Handball	Basketball	Tennis	Track & Field	Marathon	Triathlon	Other Sports
5,150	2,129	312	830	760	420	879	670
							Cycling, Running, Martial arts (e.g., Judo, etc.)

- 447 European junior-national soccer players Germany/Netherlands/France/Spain
- 2,870 pro soccer players, 867 pro handball players
- 371 pro tennis players
- 89 Olympic champions/world champions/European champions/German champions/state champions (from all sports)

Fig. 12

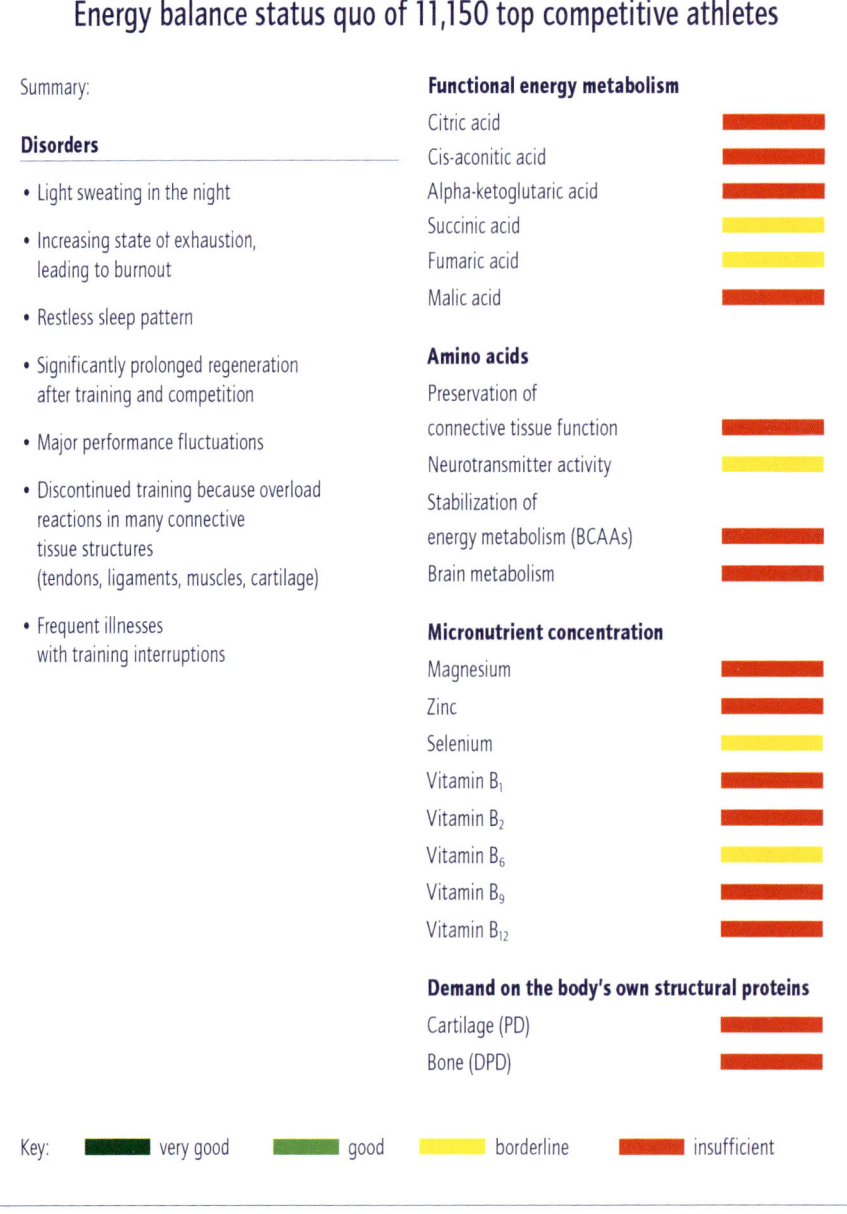

Fig. 13

INTRODUCTION

And 100% report a direct link between "Prescription for Energy" and athletic success!

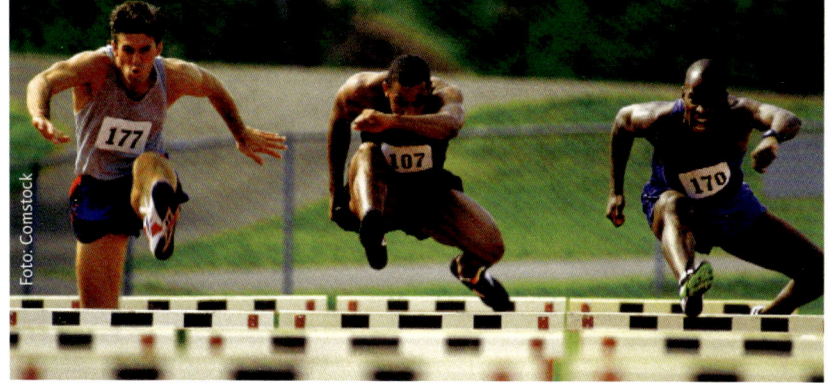

Fig. 14

First we outline the starting basis of the complex energy metabolism of these athletes in an overall layout with the aid of specially-developed blood and urine analyses (see Fig. 13).

Our tests are substantiated by the results from an anonymous survey conducted by the Cologne Sports College by order of the German Sports Aid Foundation (see Fig. 14).

The many biochemical disorders we initially detected in the 11,150 top competitive athletes can be markedly reduced after only six months of an individualized "Prescription for Optimal Energy" (see Fig. 15), albeit continued optimization potential exists after these six months. The positive changes in the energy metabolism show definite links between an optimal energy balance and the athletes' performance capacity.

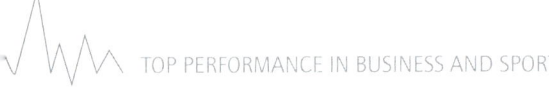

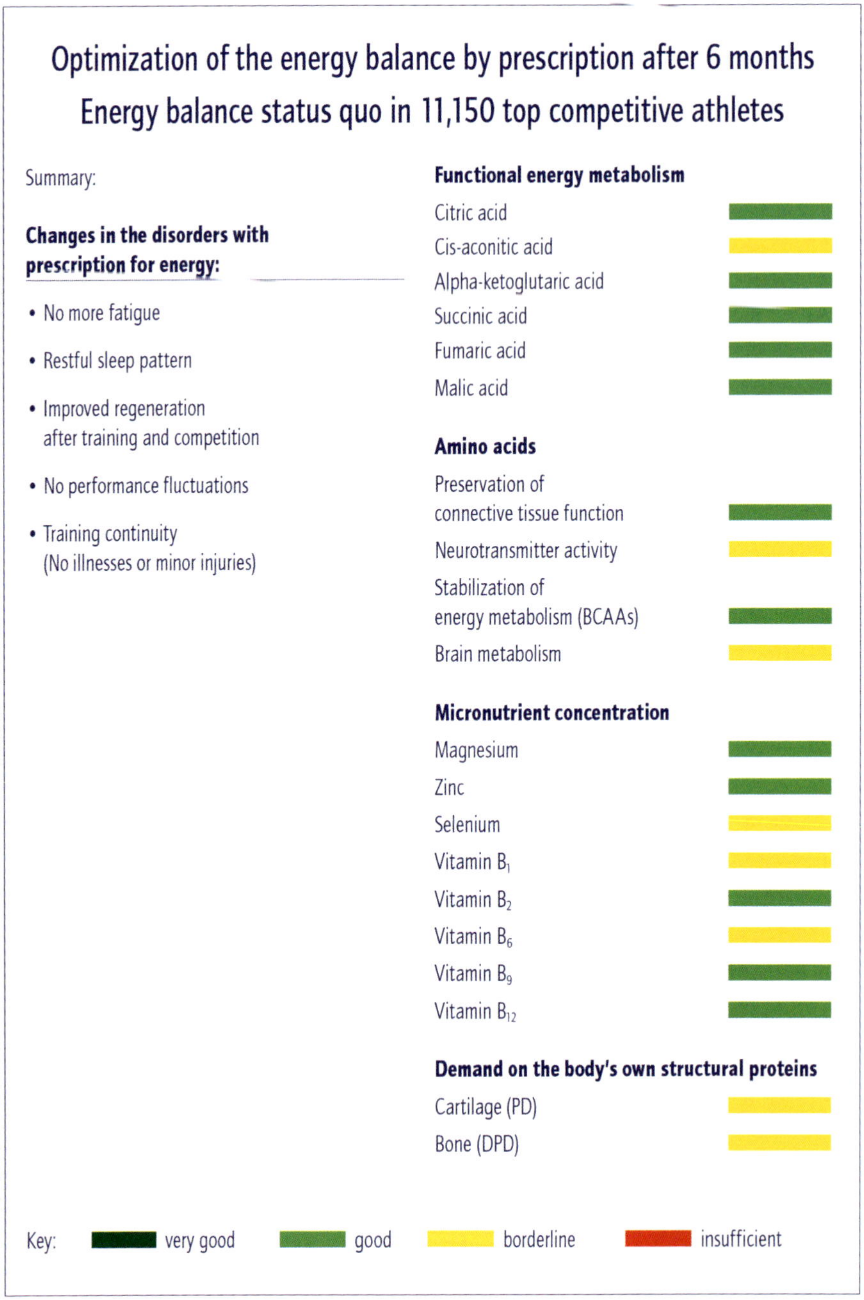

Optimization of the energy balance by prescription after 6 months
Energy balance status quo in 11,150 top competitive athletes

Summary:

Changes in the disorders with prescription for energy:

- No more fatigue
- Restful sleep pattern
- Improved regeneration after training and competition
- No performance fluctuations
- Training continuity (No illnesses or minor injuries)

Functional energy metabolism

Citric acid	🟩 very good
Cis-aconitic acid	🟨 borderline
Alpha-ketoglutaric acid	🟩 very good
Succinic acid	🟩 very good
Fumaric acid	🟩 very good
Malic acid	🟩 very good

Amino acids

Preservation of connective tissue function	🟩 very good
Neurotransmitter activity	🟨 borderline
Stabilization of energy metabolism (BCAAs)	🟩 very good
Brain metabolism	🟨 borderline

Micronutrient concentration

Magnesium	🟩 very good
Zinc	🟩 very good
Selenium	🟨 borderline
Vitamin B_1	🟨 borderline
Vitamin B_2	🟩 very good
Vitamin B_6	🟨 borderline
Vitamin B_9	🟩 very good
Vitamin B_{12}	🟩 very good

Demand on the body's own structural proteins

Cartilage (PD)	🟨 borderline
Bone (DPD)	🟨 borderline

Key: 🟩 very good　🟢 good　🟨 borderline　🟥 insufficient

Fig. 15

LONG-TERM SUCCESSES

Optimization and progression of the energy metabolism in 2,150 top competitive athletes over a period of six years (2006-2012) via an optimal energy intake by prescription (see pg. 36) shows how initial deficiencies normalize in subsequent years. The many measurements of the energy metabolism took place twice a year along with the appropriate adjustment to the individualized prescription. Further details regarding the many components of the prescription can be found in the example cases (see chapters 7.2 and 7.3).

Many international elite athletes (Olympic champions, world champions, European champions, German champions) have benefitted for years from Prescription for Energy and are thereby able to train intensely at a higher level and can tap into their full potential during competitions. The self-reports from 2,150 top competitive athletes shows how the Prescription for Energy concept has progressed in all kinds of sports over the course of six years based on the athletes' subjective feelings. This progression in the individual athletes can also be scientifically proven with the individual case reports.

In the beginning, we were skeptical, but after six weeks we were already able to:

- Train and play at a higher performance level
- Regenerate more quickly after training and competing
- Feel subjectively stronger while training and competing
- Verifiably improved immune system, and reduced illness rate
- Enjoyed a subjective feeling of strength and endurance (optimal mental and physical readiness to perform)

Our conclusion: We were able to achieve an extreme improvement in physical performance capacity with the individualized prescriptions.

RESULTS FROM THE INDIVIDUAL ANALYSES AND THEIR PROGRESSION VIA PRESCRIPTION FOR OPTIMAL ENERGY IN 2,150 TOP COMPETITIVE ATHLETES

Functional energy metabolism

Where the dark blue bars meets the red bar, we can see impairment in the activity of certain enzymes (accelerate chemical processes) that results in a verifiable decrease in energy production. Normalization or economization of the metabolism can be achieved with an individualized energy intake by prescription and can be verifiably detected over a period of six years.

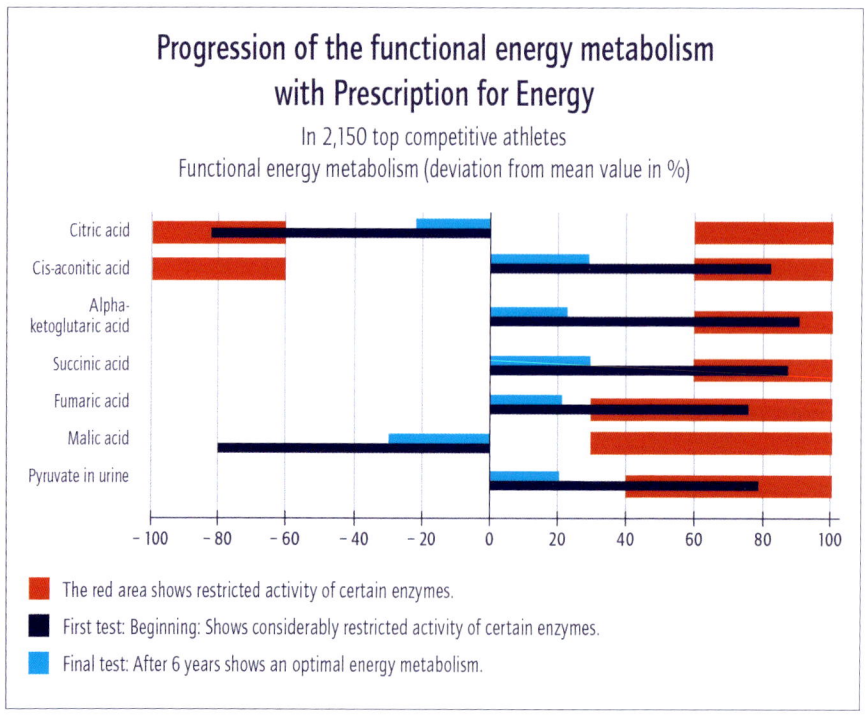

Fig. 16

Amino acids

Increasing exhaustion, poor regeneration, and performance fluctuations are often a result of biochemical disturbances caused by dificiencies in various amino acids that can lead to many disorders.

INTRODUCTION

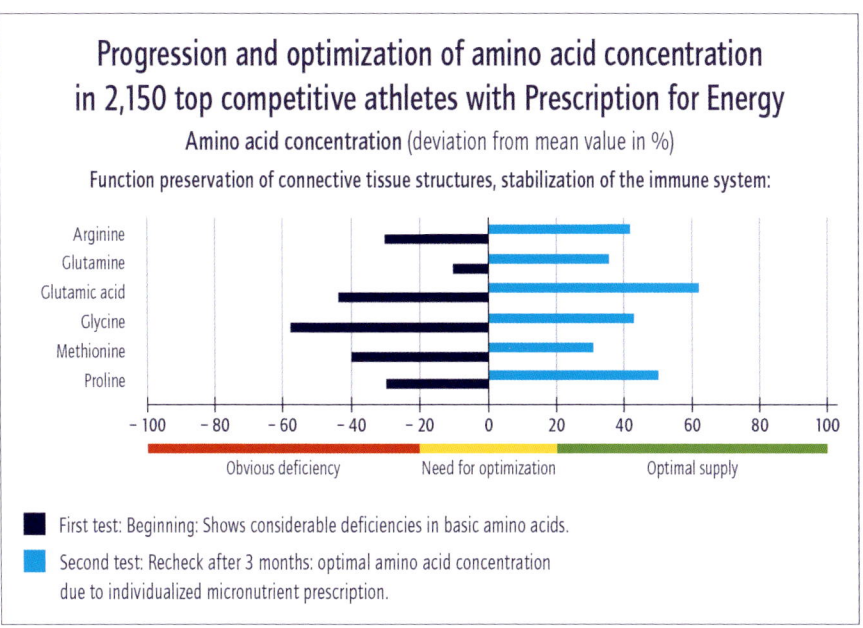

Fig. 17

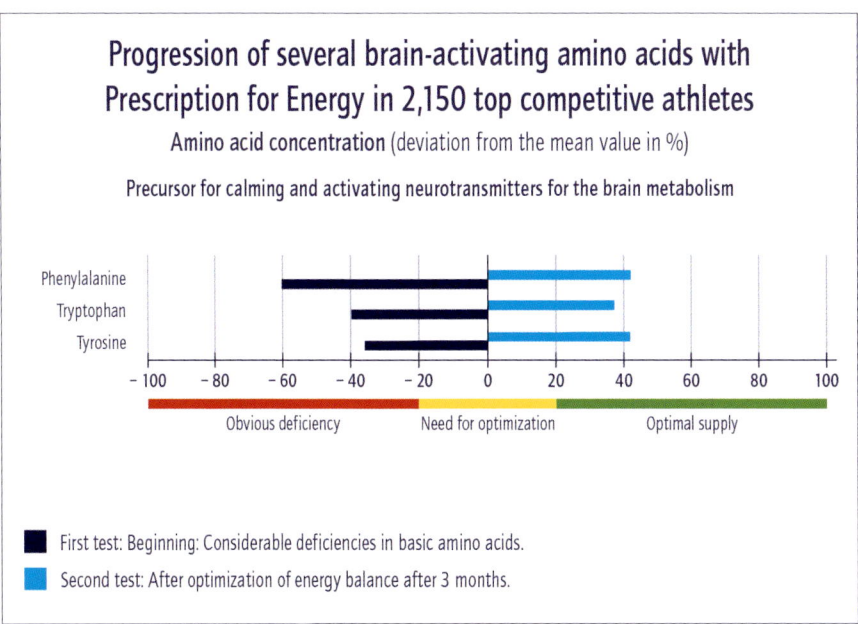

Fig. 18

The demand on connective tissue structures (tendons, ligaments, muscles, cartilage) in particular shows that in top competitive athletes, amino acid concentrations above +20% of the mean value verifiably connote protection from injuries as well as increased mental alertness (see chapter 7.3). This state of mental alertness is apparent in the case reports of 1,150 top competitive athletes with concentrations 20% above the mean value of brain-activating amino acids.

Intracellular micronutrient concentrations

Important biochemical mechanisms of actions of elements take place primarily on the cellular level. Determining the element concentration from the serum does not therefore provide information about cellular processes (see pg. 68). With a targeted intake of individualized Prescription for Energy the micronutrient concentration can be optimized within a year to the point where biochemical disorders in the metabolism normalize.

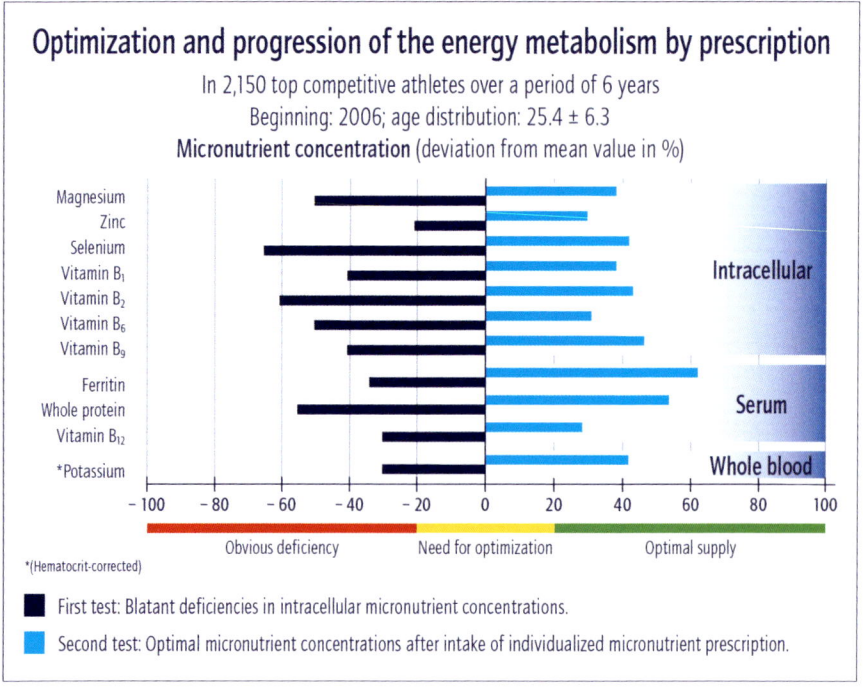

Fig. 19

Demand on the body's own structural proteins (pyridine crosslinks)

A sufficient energy intake prevents excessive demand on the body's own structural proteins and is fundamentally important to the preservation of connective tissue (tendons, ligaments, muscles, cartilage) function. Fig. 20 shows how the use of Prescription for Energy results in a noticeably decreased demand on the body's own structural proteins after just six months.

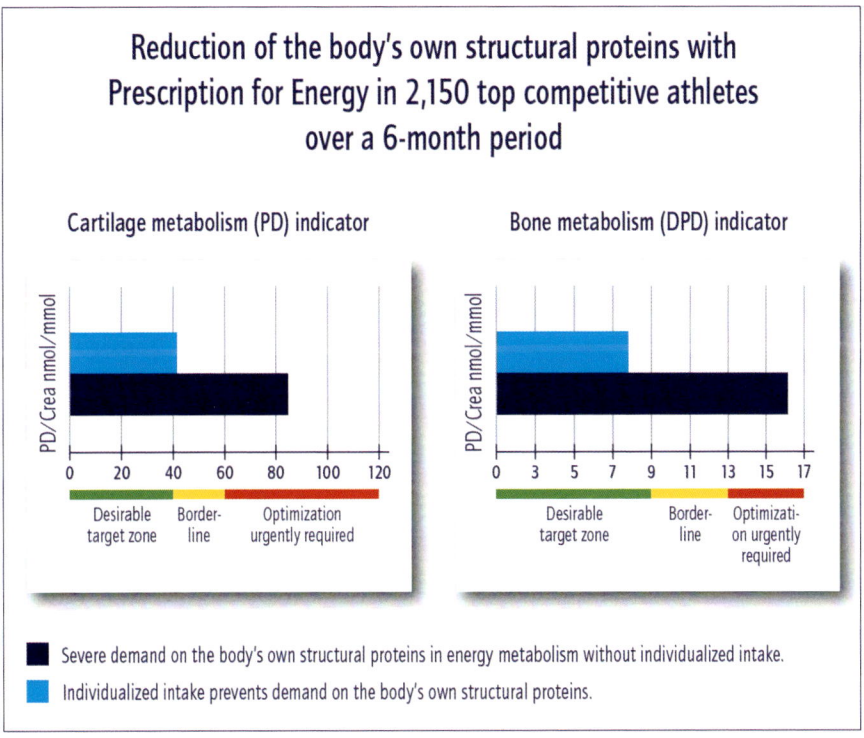

Fig. 20

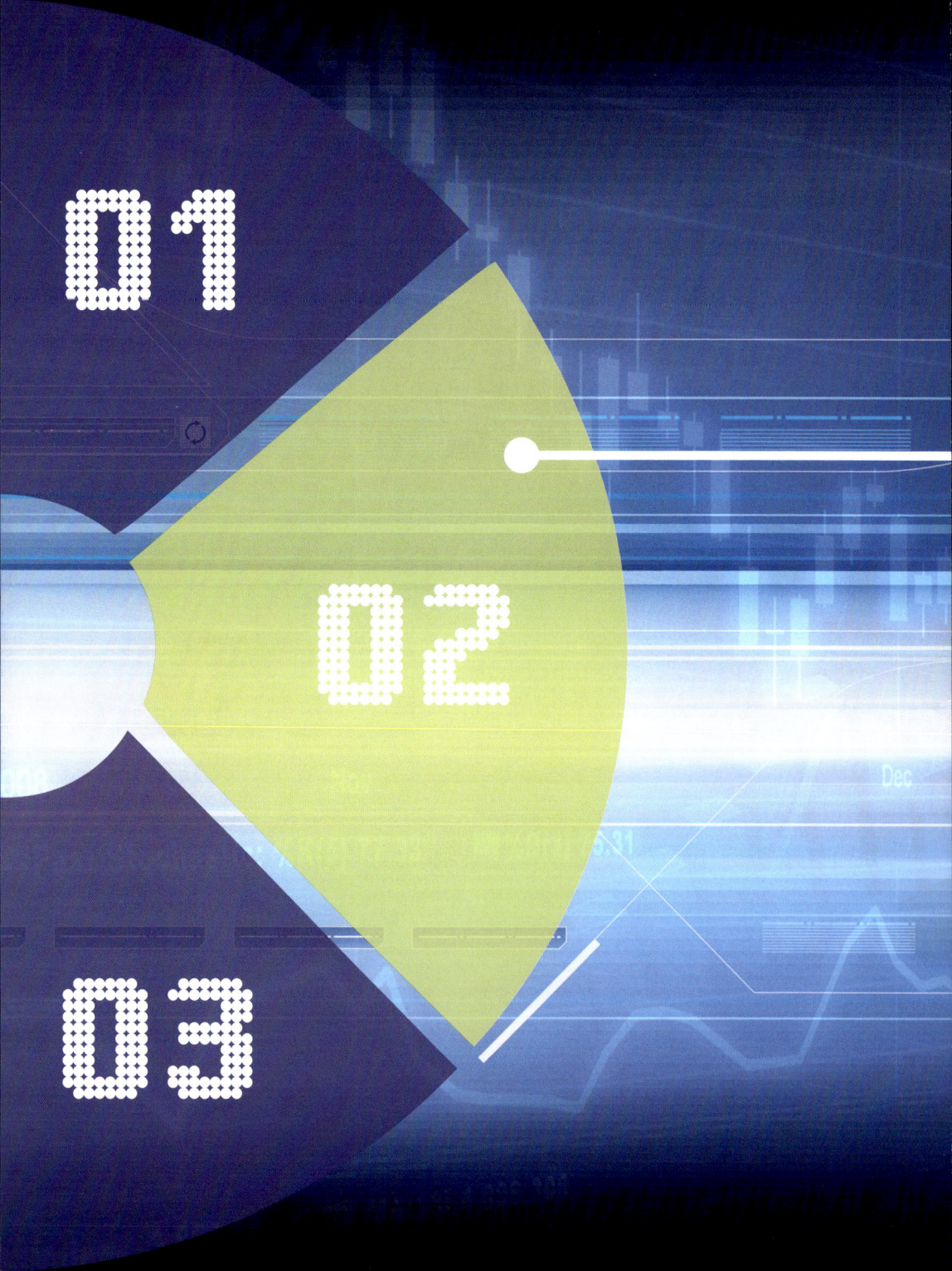

Internal and External Energy: Living a Balanced Life

2 INTERNAL AND EXTERNAL ENERGY: LIVING A BALANCED LIFE

2.1 GENERAL ASPECTS OF OUR ENERGY BALANCE

INNER CONTENTMENT: THE ENERGY SUPPLIER

Quality of life, inner contentment, fulfilling relationships with partners and family, professional success, and lots of fun and happy times socializing with friends ensure optimal energy. But there is a common denominator that constitutes the prerequisite for all positive energy flow: health, overall physical, mental, and spiritual well-being that makes it possible to pursue and achieve your individual goals.

PERSONAL RESPONSIBILITY IS GOOD—BUT NOT ALWAYS EASY

Actually life is good! For years, our life expectancy has been steadily going up, hardly anyone in the industrialized world suffers from hunger, and many illnesses that our ancestors had to suffer helplessly today can be effectively treated with modern medicine. And still few people feel as though their life is heaven on earth. Good health is much more than an extension of life. The dramatic increase in chronic fatigue syndrome to the en vogue expression *burnout* causes more and more people to be professionally marginalized. In addition, there are new illnesses on the rise that spring from today's life style: cardiovascular and metabolic diseases or damages to bones and joints caused by obesity or inappropriate physical stress.

And with respect to nutrition, our confidence has been shaken by constant bad news about pollution loads or decreasing nutrient density in our food.

WHAT DAMPENS OUR WELLBEING

Recent findings show that 1 in 2 German citizens, regardless of age, complains about different disorders: He is chronically fatigued, has frequent illnesses, trouble concentrating, suffers from a lack of motivation, headaches, exhaustion, etc.

While in 2,000, only 70 in 1,000 employees exhibited symptoms of exhaustion, today that number has quintupled to 370 out of 1,000 employees in German companies. Out of 10,270 executives (entrepreneurs, executive managers, executive staff), 70% exhibit increasing symptoms of exhaustion (see pg. 18, fig. 1). Out of 11,150 top competitive athletes tested by SALUTO, 69% lack mental alertness (see pg. 30, fig. 10). Top athletes exhibit considerable performance fluctuations and are unable to meet their full potential because of smaller injuries (see pg. 30, 31).

INCREASING STRESSORS
DISRUPT THE BRAIN'S BIOCHEMICAL EQUILIBRIUM

These various overload reactions and associated disorders can be prevented with an optimal energy intake. The brain reacts based on biochemical principles. When specific substances are lacking, certain functional sequences can no longer proceed optimally, resulting in premature exhaustion.

The top athlete suffers from a sharp decline in form and does not meet his potential. The manager feels burned out, the woman with the double burden of job and family is overwhelmed, and the pensioner/retiree suffers from various disorders. All too often therapists are unable to find an adequate explanation for the causes. Here an optimal energy intake can verifiably help.

OPTIMAL ENERGY WITH EARLY AND ACCURATE DIAGNOSTICS

The increasingly faster pace of professional life and the lack of recovery time are being debated as the causes for the massive increase in these disorders. Sensory overload from modern media and constant reachability are also factors. Previous treatment approaches with medications as well as psychotherapy did little to alleviate these disorders and barely reduced the amount of disability leave. Findings from our long-time experience in the area of prevention show that timely compensation for deficient micronutrients can verifiably improve the brain metabolism, performance capacity, and thus general well-being of the individual. People, who benefit from these findings today are, free of many ailments, and can achieve quality of life with an optimized energy balance. All of our parameters are archived in a one-of-a-kind data bank and help us in our analysis and evaluation of your energy requirements.

2.2 FIT INSTEAD OF EXHAUSTED: THE PATH TO INCREASED ENERGY

MORE ENERGY WITH MODERATE EXERCISE

Overall interest in health topics by executives and highly-committed professionals is bigger than ever. Ten years ago, many of these people went to fitness studios. But all too often, joining up was the result of a heroic decision with not much consequence. Joining and then exercising regularly are two very different things. And so it happened that a majority of supposed exercisers were actually fitness or sports club members on paper only.

Others literally seek out the challenge, but trying to balance professional life with top athletic achievement is not always the best model. Our experience in recent years shows that executives, particuularly, who have extremely demanding jobs seek a questionable athletic equivalent. Their motto is, "More helps more!" Far from it! Using such little time so intensively is not the right maxim here. We will show you how to really stay fit (see pg. 112-121).

BEING RELAXED AND ENJOYING LIFE

Everything works better when we are relaxed. "Strength lies in calmness!" Of course it does, but how do we find calmness when there is chaos? The psyche wants to be cared for, too, so daily demands won't get the best of us. There are some active strategies for stress reduction. Each person should find out which of these strategies are best for him. Relaxation can be learned. See chapter 5.3 for more detailed information.

HEALTHY AND DEEP SLEEP AS AN ENERGY SOURCE

Healthy and deep sleep can verifiably strengthen the immune system and prevent increasing exhaustion long-term. How much sleep does a person need? Find out on pg. 145, chapter 5.4, how performance capacity can be preserved with optimal sleep systems.

2.3 DIGRESSION: THE COMPLEX ENERGY SYSTEM

BRIEF CHARACTERIZATION OF ANABOLISM

The energy necessary for the previously mentioned functions in the cells is obtained through incremental oxidation of the following nutrients:

- Sugar, e.g. dextrose (glucose)
- Fats (especially fatty acids)
- Proteins (amino acids)

Based on newer research, proteins are increasingly used for energy production during intense and long workouts. Here there is the risk of long-term depletion of important protein structures, which are then insufficiently available to build up many connective tissue structures (tendons, ligaments, muscles, cartilage) and the immune system.

The biological oxidations are similar to burning processes that take place without flames and at relatively low temperatures. Oxidation generally refers to the release of electrons (e-). In the process high-energy nutrients turn into low-energy compounds, such as urea, CO_2, and H_2O.

Principles of energy supply
in the skeletal muscles during physical activity

During physical stress in sports, the energy demand goes up due to the energy-requiring muscle contractions. Depending on the type and intensity of the workload, this increased energy turnover can be considerably higher than the rest requirement. Thus the maximum energy requirement increase per time unit of an athlete running at top speed is more than thousand fold. In addition, to that the energy requirement increase during a short distance sprint starts suddenly and already ends after 10-20 seconds.

Here, too, the principle that during oxidative breakdown of nutrients incrementally released energy is not directly transported to the energy-requiring cellular processes, but rather is stored in the high-energy phosphate compounds, is actualized. The two most important high-energy phosphate compounds are:

- *ATP* (adenosine triphosphate)
- *CP* (creatine phosphate)

The entire amount of energy from both high-energy compounds is enough for about 20 maximum muscle contractions (approximately 6-10 sec.). But since maximum physical effort must be generated with considerably more muscle contractions, chemical reactions must take place in the active muscle cells that supply energy to replenish the ATP and CP energy stores. The energy resupply occurs via biological oxidation of nutrients. There are two principle types of biological oxidation of nutrients:

- *aerobic oxidation* of nutrients with oxygen use and
- *anaerobic oxidation* of carbohydrates (primarily glucose) without oxygen.

Aerobic oxidation

Aerobic oxidation tales place in the mitochondria. To this purpose, oxygen and pyruvate (pyruvic acid) must be transported to the mitochondria. Conversely, the generated ATP as well as the formed CO_2 and H_2O leave the mitochondria.

The mitochondria are the energy suppliers to the cells and are also referred to as *power stations*. Nutrients like sugar and fat that find their way to the cells are burned in the mitochondria with the help of oxygen. Similar to the cell nucleus, the mitochondria are also surrounded by a double membrane. The fluid in between the layers can be compared to the extracellular fluid that is present between the individual cells. Their inner membrane is largely unfolded and thus offers a large surface area. The mitochondria are long threads that move in a circular or winding motion. They are present in varying numbers in all cells with the exception of red blood cells (erythrocytes).

Aerobic oxidation takes place in enzyme-driven steps, which in turn consist of multiple reaction intervals. When looking at the dextrose, glycogen, stored in the muscle cell, we can differentiate different breakdown levels. However, we will forgo a detailed description. Depending on energy demand, the enzyme-driven steps of the aerobic energy supply (activation of acetic acid, citric acid cycle, and respiratory chain) are partially accelerated or slowed down via complicated reactions. If, for instance, there is a lack of magnesium, certain progressions in the endurance area cannot optimally take place.

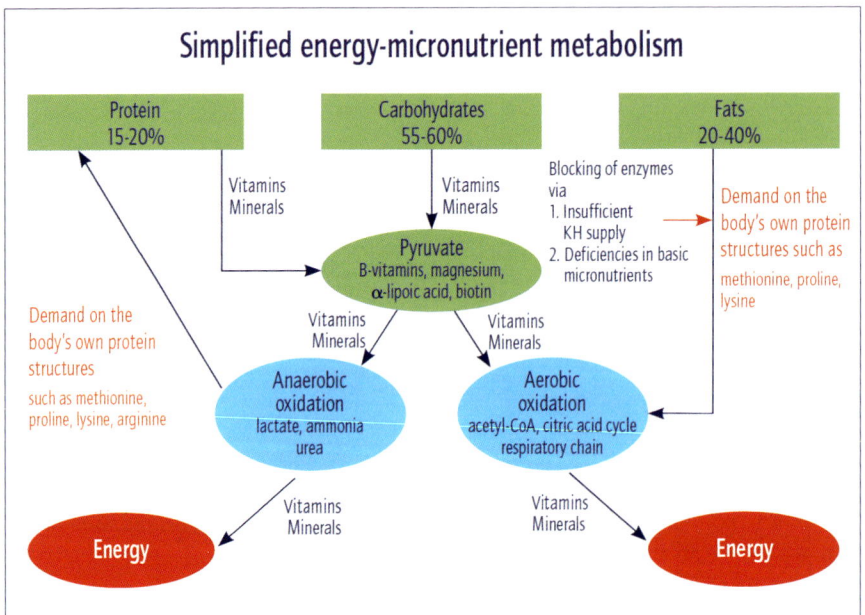

Fig. 21

Conclusion: Micronutrient (vitamins, minerals, trace elements) deficiencies during the energy supply of the carbohydrate and fat metabolism can lead to an enzyme blockage. The energy is then supplied by the body's own amino acids, which are then no longer sufficiently available for the important connective tissue structures (ligaments, tendons, cartilage).

Anaerobic oxidation

The largest portion of the energy requirement by far is supplied during physical exertion, especially during extended periods of physical exertion, via aerobic oxidation of nutrients. The second type of energy supply, *anaerobic oxidation*, is employed when the current energy requirement cannot be met via aerobic oxidation. During anaerobic oxidation, the energy is supplied from glucose that is broken down in a complex manner. Heavy lactate formation inevitably leads to muscle fatigue, and the organism is forced to reduce or completely discontinue activity.

The enzymes involved in anaerobic oxidation (glycolysis) are located in the cell plasma (sarcoplasm). Thus the anaerobic energy supply takes place in close proximity to the myofibrils in the muscle cell. Previously the assumption was that only 15% of the forming lactate was converted back to glucose in the liver with the use of energy. But many scientists from different spheres of knowledge vehemently challenge this. They believe that this percentage is much higher and can also take place from the amino acids.

While the energy from the high-energy phosphates is only sufficient for a maximum workload duration of 6 sec., during an anaerobic—lactic acid energy supply, this duration is about 60 sec. and increases to 60 min. during aerobic energy supply from glycogen. Fatty acids as aerobic energy suppliers increase the maximum workload duration to considerably longer than 60 min. An inadequate replenishment of glycogen stores in the liver and musculature because of severe micronutrient deficiencies after intense exertion very quickly leads to short-term activation of the body's own amino acids, which are then no longer sufficiently available to build up the connective tissue of ligaments, tendons, and cartilage structures.

2.4 PHYSICAL AND MENTAL PERFORMANCE CAPACITY AND THE ROLE OF MICRONUTRIENTS IN THE ENERGY METABOLISM

Thiamine (B_1), riboflavin (B_2), aniacin (B_3), and pantothenic acid are used within the scope of energy supply. Folic acid (B_9) and vitamin B_{12} are needed for the production of new red blood cells (erythrocytes). Vitamin E acts as an antioxidant, especially for cell membranes and muscle fibers. Vitamin C supports the production of adrenaline. Niacin possibly inhibits free-fatty acid release. Vitamin B_1, B_6, and B_{12} are involved in the formation of neurotransmitters in the brain, which play an important role in fatiguing and recovery processes. If, for instance, there is a lack of certain amino acids and vitamins, the energy metabolism is only able to work with "a foot on the brake."

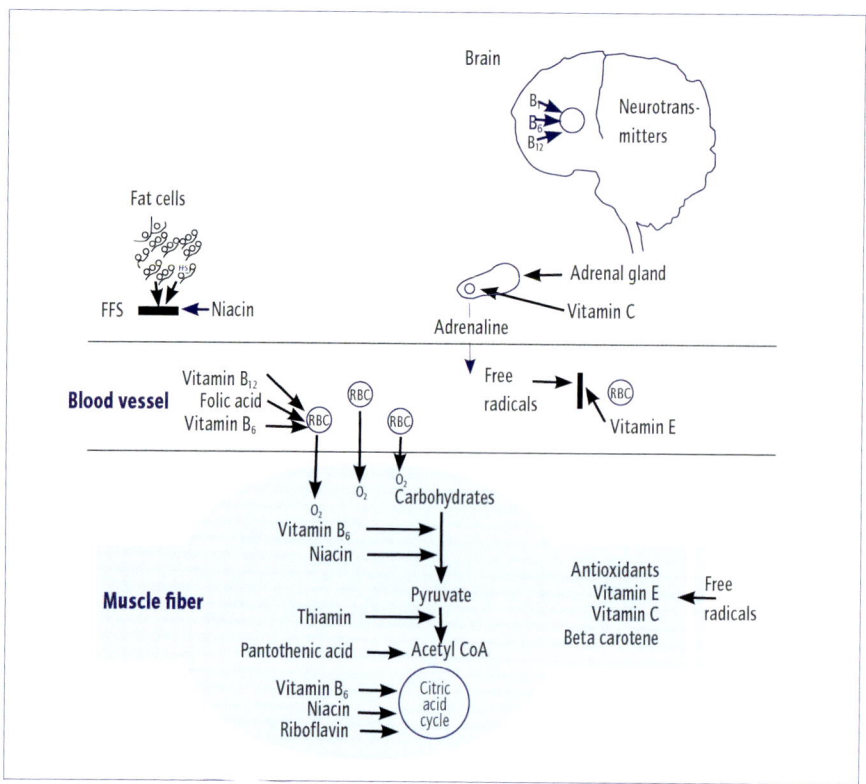

Fig. 22: Excerpt from the Sports Encyclopedia, German Medical Publishing

Impaired activity of certain enzymes in the energy metabolism in executives and athletes verifiably results in biochemical disruptions that lead to a significantly reduced energy production, and can trigger a number of disorders (see pg. 22, fig. 4). Results show, for instance, that considerable functional impairment of the energy metabolism exists in 4,150 executives as a result of existing cellular micronutrient deficiencies. Top competitive athletes show similar values analogous to these results (see pg. 33, fig. 14).

"Humans don't get sick because the body lacks medicine, but because biochemical disturbances occur in the body that are not deteced and corrected!"

B. Kuklinski, environmental and nutritional medicine specialist

Each person has an individual energy and micronutrient requirement
Our 21,420 case reports show marked deficiencies in the energy and micronutrient balance of executives and top athletes that are linked to many disorders. Today these energy and micronutrient requirements can be individually analyzed and evaluated with special diagnostics and a respective comprehensive data bank. Worldwide there are very few institutes that have access to the applicable reference data and also capture the different groups of people individually and are able to evaluate them.

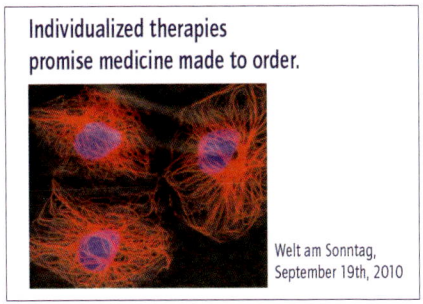

Individualized therapies promise medicine made to order.	Reality
Welt am Sonntag, September 19th, 2010	To date there are **no** physical performance data for the practical testing of clinical relevance of previous dosages. Previous dosage recommendations are derived from considerations of energy expenditure versus increased nutrient requirements. (Quote from Sportmedizin für Ärzte, 2007)

Fig. 23   Fig. 24

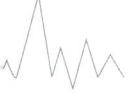

TOP PERFORMANCE IN BUSINESS AND SPORTS

Our results show the individual deviations from the mean values in percentage of comparable people in the appropriate age category (personal lifestyle, prior illnesses, athletic activity, sex). If the different groups of people are above 25% of the respective mean value, we can see mental and physical stability, and no evidence of exhaustion. The individual feels even-tempered and is extremely resilient.

A healthy diet is undeniably the basis for an equalized energy balance, but in reality, it appears to be hardly viable. Of the executives we tested (entrepreneurs, executive managers, executive staff), 70% are dissatisfied with their dietary habits. Even the 11,159 top competitive athletes, who consciously abide by the government's nutritional guidelines, show definite impairment of the energy and micronutrient balance. The consequential biochemical disorders have many causes.

The individual energy and micronutrients requirements result from the following factors:

- Lifestyle (current dietary habits)

- Athletic activity (type of sport, training volume)

- Sex

- Age

- Prior illnesses

- +20% deviation from mean values of respective group of people

2.5 THE THYROID AS REGULATOR OF THE ENERGY AND MICRONUTRIENT METABOLISM

VITALITY AND STRENGTH BY OPTIMALLY-BALANCED THYROID HORMONES

More than half of the 10,270 entrepreneurs, executives, and executive staff and 11,150 top competitive athletes tested show signs of a latent hypothyroidism that does not result in treatment suggestions based on medical expertise, but can trigger many disorders.

Iodine and selenium control thyroid function and thereby the entire energy balance. Iodine and selenium deficiency can induce an extreme thyroid problem (insomnia, anxiety, fluctuating concentration). Germany is known to be iodine deficient. In Germany, the recommended dosage of 200 µg of iodine via food including iodized salt lies at 100 µg per day. The trace element iodine is a vital component of the thyroid hormones thyroxin (T4) and triiodothyronine (T_3) and thus is essential to the entire metabolism. The thyroid's iodine-containing precursor hormone triiodothyronine is converted selenium-dependent into the active thyroid hormone (T_3).

The extraordinary importance of the thyroid hormones lies in the division and growth of all cells; the carbohydrate, protein, and fat metabolisms; the body's temperature regulation; and the energy metabolism. Any disruption in the production of thyroid hormones affects the entire organism. An inadequate iodine supply results in a drop of the thyroid hormone level in the blood. The thyroid reacts to this with increasing growth and gets larger. It attempts to balance the thyroid hormone deficiency with increased production. A visible sign is the goiter at the neck, also called *struma*.

**PRESENCE OF LATENT SYMPTOMS—
BUT UNTIL NOW WITHOUT CLINICAL RELEVANCE**

Based on our test results, more than half the executives and competitive athletes we tested show a latent hypothyroidism. Those affected initially feel a little tired, cold-sensitive, and regularly have light night sweats. After a while they appear unmotivated and only regenerate very slowly after intense exertion. We frequently see these symptoms even in young athletes. In youth athletes, this iodine deficiency is often characterized by difficulties learning and concentrating and frequent illnesses. Anyone who has these symptoms should have his iodine levels checked.

Challenging lab results on thyroid hormones (reference ranges)

Our experience from recent years and new findings from the United States show that previous reference ranges should be challenged. In "What the soul wants to eat" (Ross, 2010), physicians describe a considerably more nuanced view of previous thyroid hormones and their impact on many disorders.

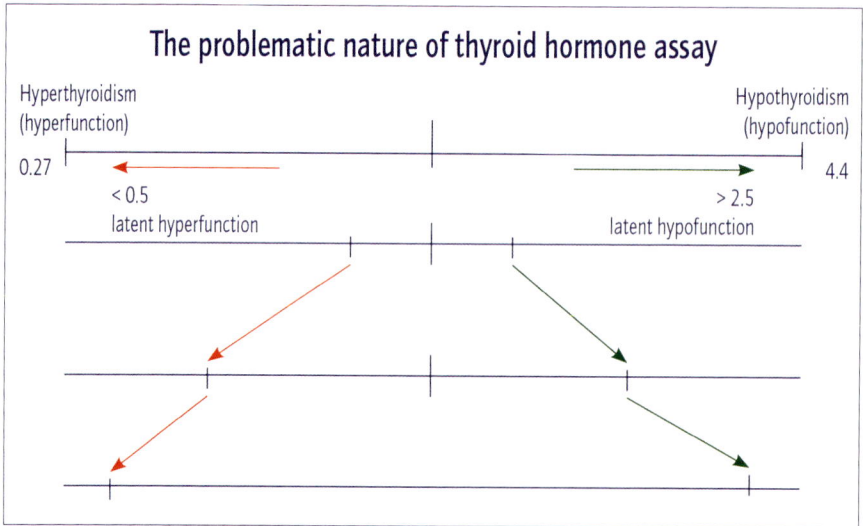

Fig. 25

In fig. 25, we can see the problem with interpreting the initial measurement of the TSH value. Based on our experience, a latent hypofunction lies at a TSH value of > 2.5 µIU/ml. It is our experience that this can already be an initial performance-diminishing factor in executives and competitive athletes. The progression of respective values over a longer period of time is pivotal here.

These should also be compared to the subjective feeling of the individuals.

Important advice

After intense exertion during training and competition, the stress-induced thyroid hormone level is often considerably higher the next morning. For this reason, thyroid hormone tests are only meaningful if no direct, intense athletic exertion took place on the previous day.

Balanced thyroid hormones

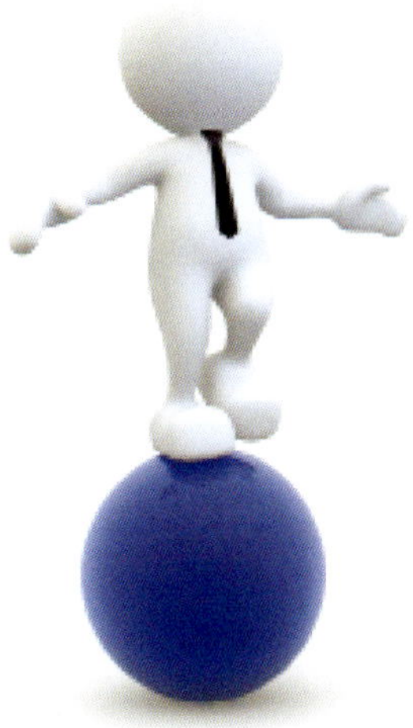

TSH- basal values 1.6-2.2 µIU/ml

- Optimal training ability
- Good mental and physical performance capacity
- Good sleep pattern
- Fast regeneration after athletic exertion

Fig. 26

The comprehensive test results from 21,420 executives and athletes show that many disorders can be corrected with a targeted iodine intake or a medication that normalizes thyroid hormone levels. TSH-basal values that were between 1.6 µIU/ml and 2.2 µIU/ml in the people tested (see fig. 26) provide no indication of the aforementioned disorders. The identification of relevant antibodies ruled out an autoimmune disease.

SALUTO Institute and our partners will continue to initiate research projects involving executives and competitive athletes with borderline thyroid hormone status and scientifically challenge previous experience.

PERMANENTLY TENSE AS A BOW STRING

Of the 11,150 executives and 10,270 competitive athletes, 15% have thyroid hormone levels that trend towards hyperfunction (hyperthyroidism), however based on a different scientific understanding: The physicians speak of a latent hyperfunction (hyperthyroidism) at TSH-basal values of < 0.5 µIU/ml. However, we have found that at THS-basal values of < 1.3 µIU/ml, a definite sympathicotony (pronounced activation of the vegetative nervous system) already exists with individual aspects of the following disorders (see fig. 27).

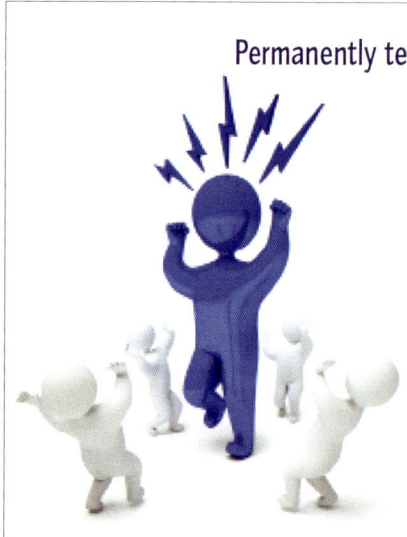

Fig. 27

Simple problem-solving approach

Depending on results from the cellular analysis, the targeted intake of iodine over the course of the day (morning, midday, evening) can verifiably "ramp down" the vegetative nervous system (also see case reports, chapters 7.2 and 7.3). If the measurement values for tryptophan were low, an appropriate intake is given in accordance with the starting situation. After four to five days, we could see a definite improvement in the sleep quality of our executives and top athletes.

SLEEPING-PILL MENTALITY

The executives and competitive athletes we tested often already show signs of a latent hypothyroidism at TSH-basal values of > 2.5 µIU/ml that caused some of the following disorders (see fig. 28) in this group of people.

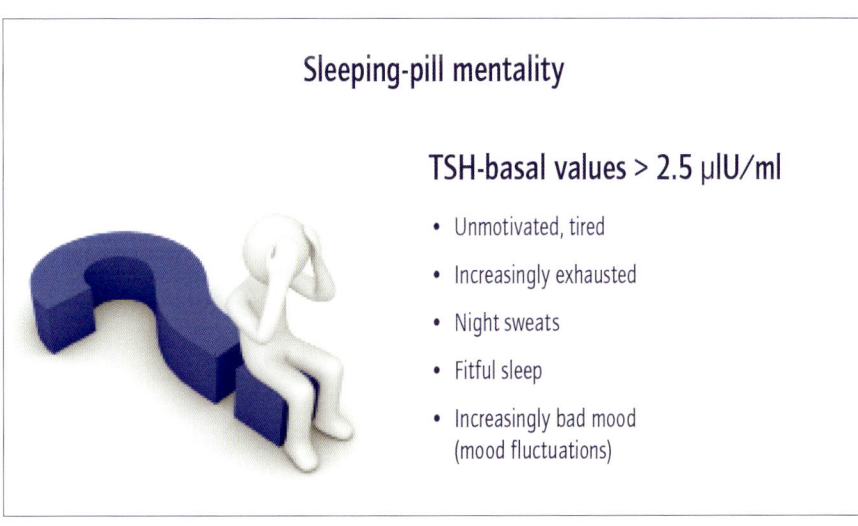

Fig. 28

These can be relieved with a targeted intake of iodine (dosage depends on thyroid hormone level) or a suitable medication (e.g., appropriate dose of thyroxin).

Based on our experience, a TSH-basal value of > 2.8 µIU/ml can result in a definite long-term impairment of physical and mental performance capacity. If we can detect this early enough using regular testing, these disorders can be avoided.

An example case: The author as subject

Example of a long-existing latent hypothyroidism (hypofunction) in the author:

I start my day every morning around 5:30 with strength training followed by 40-45 minutes of endurance training. At the age of 47, I became increasingly fatigued and unmotivated. I suddenly experienced unusual night sweats. I also experienced sudden claustrophobia in the elevator and felt increasingly depressed. I had my thyroid levels checked right away. According to the lab physicians' standards, the measurements were an acceptable value of 3.3 µIU/ml. I showed this value to a friend who is an internist and asked for his help. He told me that at my age initial hormonal changes take place that could be typical andropause symptoms. The TSH-basal value combined with the T_3 and T_4 values were within an acceptable range. During my many years of caring for athletes, I have frequently heard these same complaints. I therefore decided to practice exactly what we have already successfully done with athletes. Every morning I took 3x Jodid 100 before breakfast. After three weeks, all of the symptoms had disappeared, and after six weeks, the TSH-basal values had normalized to 1.8 µIU/ml.

IMPORTANT: AN ADEQUATE SELENIUM CONCENTRATION

Next to iodine, selenium is essential to thyroid hormone synthesis. When there is an iodine deficiency in the thyroid, additional toxic hydroperoxides form that are rendered harmless by selenium-containing glutathione peroxidase. Thyroid disorders can also result from a selenium deficiency. When there is a lack of selenium the active thyroid hormone triiodothyronine (T_3) cannot be formed. Thus a thyroid hypofunction cannot only be caused by iodine but also selenium deficiency.

Selenium occurs in all of the body's cells and fluids. The highest concentrations are located in the thyroid, kidney, liver, spleen, heart, and prostate. Selenium is a functional component in many enzymes and proteins. Germany and many other countries count among Europe's selenium-poor regions. Even with a balanced diet, an adult gets barely more than 45 µIU/ml per day since our food usually contains little selenium. Good sources of selenium are seafood, innards, green tee, and Brazil nuts.

We were able to detect blatant cellular deficiencies in the competitive athletes we tested. A good selenium status has a positive effect on immunological stability, regeneration ability, and stress tolerance. An adequately high selenium status requires a daily intake of approximately 1.5-2 µIU/ml selenium per kg of body weight. A reasonable intake is determined by the individual cellular selenium status. A long-term intake higher than 200 µIU/ml selenium can cause toxic reactions. A prior analysis of the cellular selenium concentration is therefore recommended. This can be followed by a targeted intake.

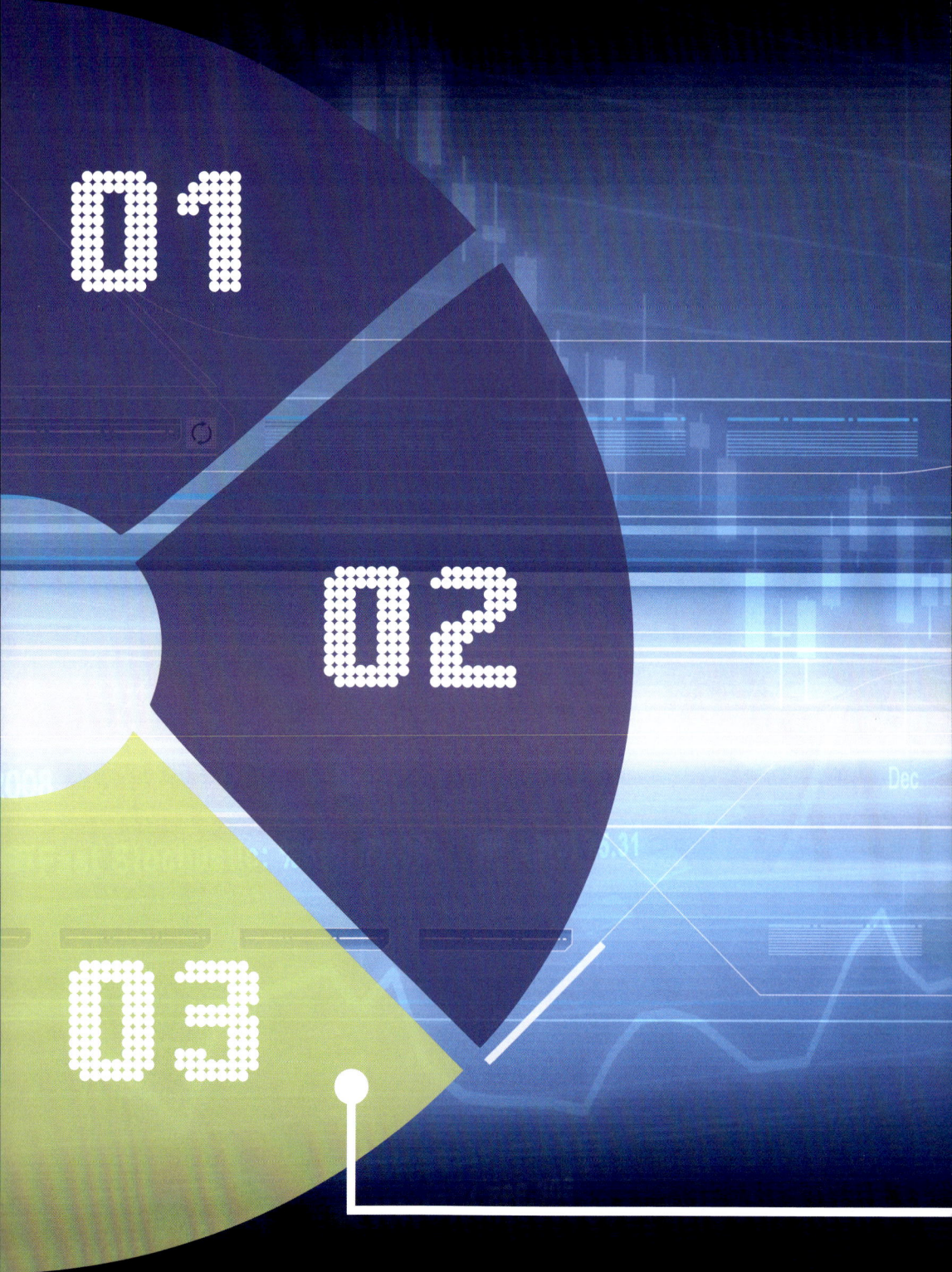

YOU ARE WHAT YOU EAT: ASPECTS OF NUTRITION PHYSIOLOGY

3 YOU ARE WHAT YOU EAT: ASPECTS OF NUTRITION PHYSIOLOGY

3.1 FUNCTIONAL ENERGY METABOLISM DISORDERS DUE TO MICRONUTRIENT DEFICIENCIES IN EXECUTIVES AND COMPETITIVE ATHLETES

Vital, fit, and productive for as long as possible, that is what executives (entrepreneurs, executive managers, executive staff) as well as competitive athletes wish for. Surely everyone is aware of the close relationship between nutrition, brain metabolism, immune system, and performance capacity. Some people may wonder why they don't feel great or aren't productive in spite of a good diet. In this chapter we will reveal what are to some extent surprising correlations and make a case for the necessary and targeted intake of vital micronutrient substances.

MICRONUTRIENT DEFICIENCY:
THE REGULATORS OF THE ENERGY SYSTEM ARE OFTEN UNKNOWN

According to a recent nutrition report by the DGE (German Nutrition Society) and statements from renowned nutrition scientists, sports scientists, and sports physicians, an additional intake of vital micronutrient substances is unnecessary and should be declined as long the individual had a balanced diet (with the exception of fluoride, iodine, and folic acid).

While studying entrepreneurs, executives, executive staff, and top athletes, we have learned differently. Only with a comprehensive analysis of the functional energy metabolism (see pg. 84-86), intracellular micronutrients (see pg. 87), amino acids (see pg. 89-90), and several other parameters can prevailing energy and micronutrient requirements of the individual person be analyzed.

Fig. 29 shows which serious impairments to the activity of certain enzymes in the energy metabolism can be detected in 1,150 executives.

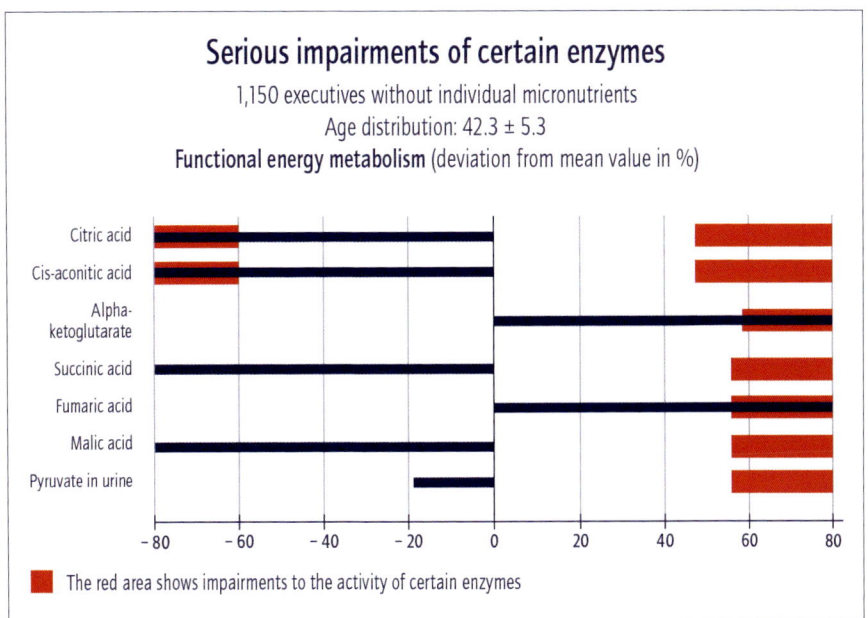

Fig. 29

3.2 THE ENGINE CANNOT RUN WITHOUT FUEL

An adequate supply of minerals and trace elements is absolutely necessary for the preservation of vital functions. Zinc, selenium, magnesium, and all the B-vitamins (a.o. B_1, B_2, B_6, B_{12}) are esprcially instrumental in a number of physiological processes of the cellular metabolism, cell division, stability, the energy metabolism, and the immune response.

Based on our latest findings, micronutrient deficiency in people with lots of professional responsibility can result in a number of long-term health problems in the form of increasing chronic fatigue syndrome with impaired cognitive performance. Competitive athletes significantly increase the risk of injury because of premature demands on the body's own structural proteins that represent an important basis for continuity of training and competing.

The results from 10,270 entrepreneurs, executives, executive staff as well as 11,150 top competitive athletes reveal that the functional energy metabolism shows impairments to the activity of certain enzymes (also see chapter 1.3 and chapter 1.4). This impairments result from cellular micronutrient deficiencies in nearly all areas, and have caused many disorders. This primarily affects people who are exposed to increasing amounts of stress.

Our own studies (e.g., clinical studies) and projects in recent years document that even with a balanced diet (according to government criteria). A severe intracellular micronutrient deficiency is detected that cannot be adequately remedied without a targeted intake of micronutrients. Here we must particularly refer to the specific cellular measurement and diagnostics of these deficiencies. In Europe there are very few laboratories that conduct these comprehensive functional analyses of the energy metabolism as well as cellular micronutrient testing and have access to a sufficiently large data bank.

ACCURATE ENERGY AND MICRONUTRIENT DIAGNOSTICS IS THE ALPHA AND OMEGA

Functional energy metabolism

A brief digression on the functional energy metabolism: The citric acid cycle forms the central switch point for the entire metabolism. It is where the breakdown of carbohydrates, fats, and proteins takes place. A deficiency in basic micronutrients (amino acids, vitamins, minerals, trace elements) results in a disruption in the "power stations" of the cells (mitochondrial dysfunction). Different metabolic products are measured here. An elevation or drop in measured substances indicates certain problems in the energy metabolism and is linked to a reduction in energy production.

The results from 4,150 executives (entrepreneurs, executive managers, executive staff) initially show definite impairment in the activity of certain enzymes in the functional energy metabolism (see fig. 4, pg. 22). An optimization of the functional energy metabolism with the individualized intake (Prescription for Energy) over a period of five years can be seen in fig. 6, pg. 24 and fig. 8, pg. 28. Additional details can be found in chapters 7.2 and 7.3.

3.3 THE COMPONENTS OF BLOOD

In a way, blood is the body's liquid transportation web or circulation assistant. Its job is to supply each cell with vital things, such as fuel from food, oxygen, vitamins, hormones, and heat, and to discharge end products of metabolism as well as heat from each cell.

The total amount of circulating blood in the human body is approximately 8% of body weight. A person weighing 80 kg thus has 6.4 l of blood. Blood consists of fluid and solids; fluids are referred to as blood plasma, solids as corpuscle.

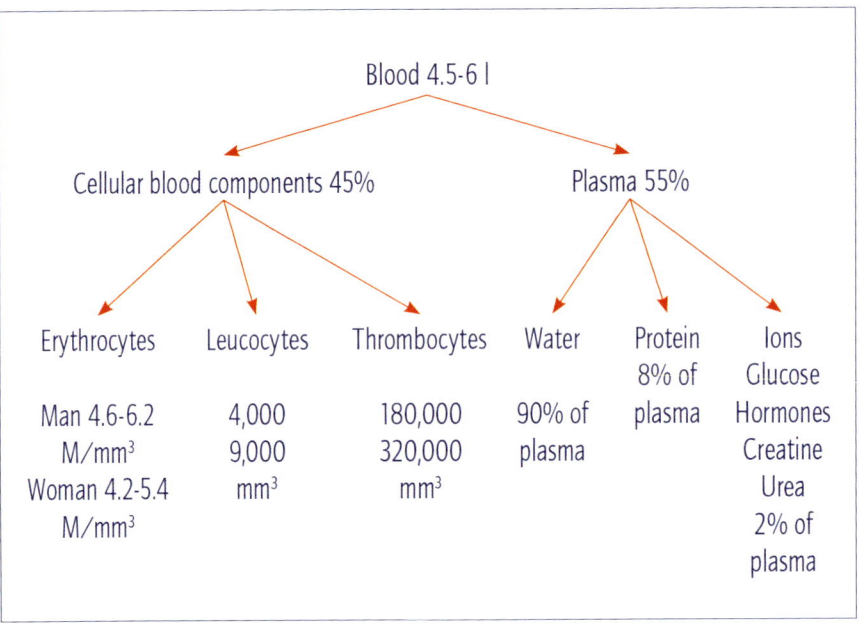

Fig. 30

Blood plasma

Blood plasma is a clear liquid. It consists of 93% water and contains substances such as common salt, carbohydrates, fats, and proteins (see fig. 30). The white blood cells (leucocytes) are the body's defense mechanism. Bacteria, viruses, funguses, and parasites that enter the body through skin injuries, respiration, or digestion are fought by blood plasma. Red blood cells (erythrocytes), at approximately 45% of the total volume, transport oxygen or carbon dioxide and contain red blood pigment (hemoglobin). During our initial years of testing, all of our blood tests were measured in the erythrocytes (intraerythrocytic) as well as in the serum. Today we measure micronutrient concentrations exclusively in the red blood cells (intraerythrocytic) because routine serum tests verifiably lack significance.

BLOOD CELLS

A long with the blood fluid (plasma), blood also contains different cells. With the exception of the lymphocytes, which also form in the lymphatic organs, all are formed in the red bone marrow (medulla ossium rubra). After some maturing time, they are then released into the blood. Their proportion of the blood varies greatly.

Red blood cells (erythrocytes) live for about three months. Then they are replaced. In a man, one cubic mm contains approximately 5 million erythrocytes, in a woman, approximately 4.5 million. Their primary purpose is to transport oxygen from the pulmonary alveoli to the organs, as well as to transport carbon dioxide back to the pulmonary alveoli from the tissue.

There are between 4,000 and 9,000 white blood cells (leucocytes) per cubic mm in the blood. The number of different white blood cells varies in the course of life and during illnesses. Leucocytes also include lymphocytes, granulocytes, and monocytes that can be seen within a differential blood count. The life span of leucocytes can span from a few hours to several years.

There are between 180,000-320,000 blood platelets (thrombocytes) per cubic mm. They are particularly important in the clotting of blood because they seal the vessel walls after an injury. Thrombocytes have a life span of 5-10 days.

Vitamins and trace elements are usually measured in the blood serum if measured at all, but not intracellular (see fig. 31). With respect to the cell's actual micronutrient supply, blood serum measurements are not diagnostically conclusive. Here a drop in the values is only noticeable when characteristic deficiency symptoms or even tissue and organ damage occurs. But latent shortages may have existed for some time without a visible acute health problem.

Blood is the transportation medium. The concentration of minerals, trace elements, and other micronutrients depends heavily on the recent absorption of these substances (e.g., through food). Routine blood tests are done on the serum level where red and white blood cells are no longer present. Thus they provide extracellular values (extracellular = outside the cells; opposite = intracellular). Elements with primarily intracellular concentrations, such as potassium, magnesium, zinc, selenium, and the B vitamins (B_1, B_2, B_6, B_{12}) cannot be captured like this. Determining of elements in serum thus does not yield reliable conclusions as to the mineral, vitamin, and trace element balance.

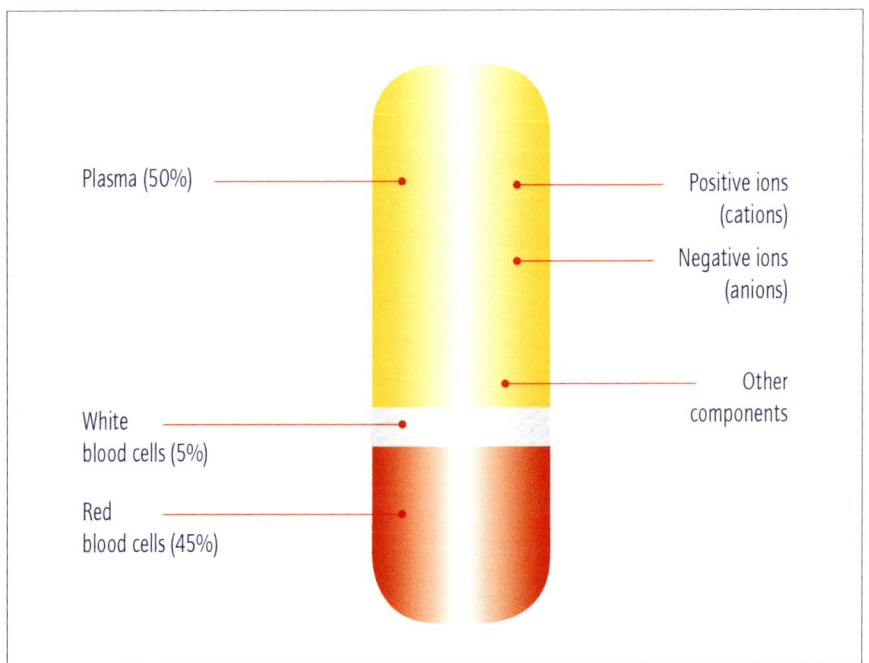

Fig. 31

Important biochemical action mechanisms of elements take place primarily on the cellular level. Determination of element concentration from serum cannot offer any information on cellular processes. The exchange between extra- and intracellular space is regulated by the body's own complex mechanisms. The concentration of important elements in the serum is kept as constant as possible. If the micronutrient supply (vitamins, minerals) is not sufficient to do so, the body's own reserves are mobilized to maintain the serum level. Therefore serum deficiencies are most often detected very late or not at all. No deficiencies were detected at the serum level in 21,420 executives (entrepreneurs, executive managers, executive staff), but definite deficiencies were found at the cellular level. Once there are deficiencies at the serum levels, deficiencies would have been ascertainable via intracellular testing.

Disorders can be present for a long time and not be substantiated with routine blood tests (see fig. 32); decreasing ability to concentrate, increasing fatigue, muscle tension, all the way to allergic reactions to pollen are just a few of the many-faceted symptoms.

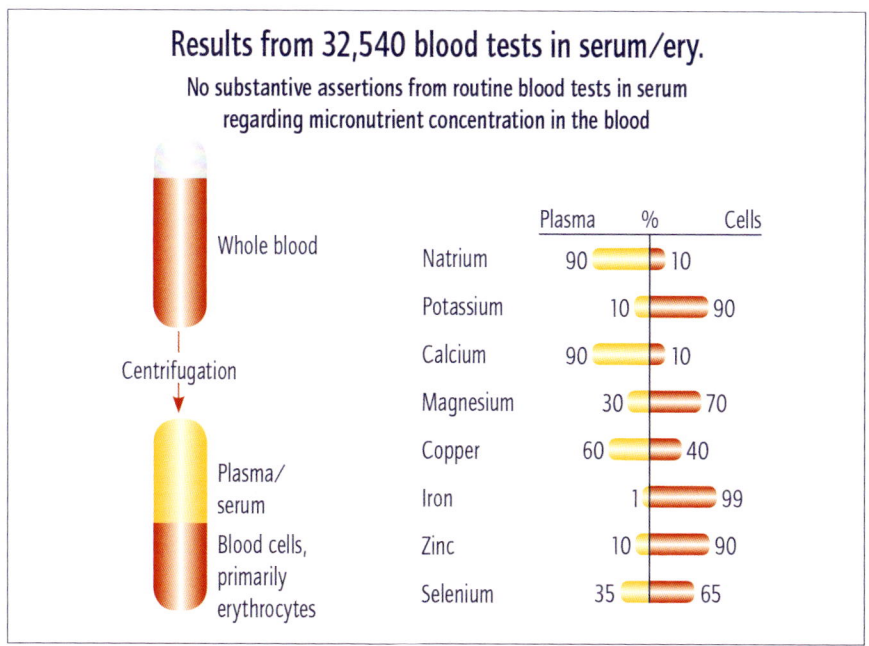

Fig. 32

But even if there are no current health problems, the goal should be not to use up one's personal resources. We detected unhappiness, insomnia, decreasing ability to concentrate, and many other disorders in the entrepreneurs, executives, and executive staff we tested. This can be avoided with timely replenishment of the cellular stores, thereby kick starting the functional energy metabolism.

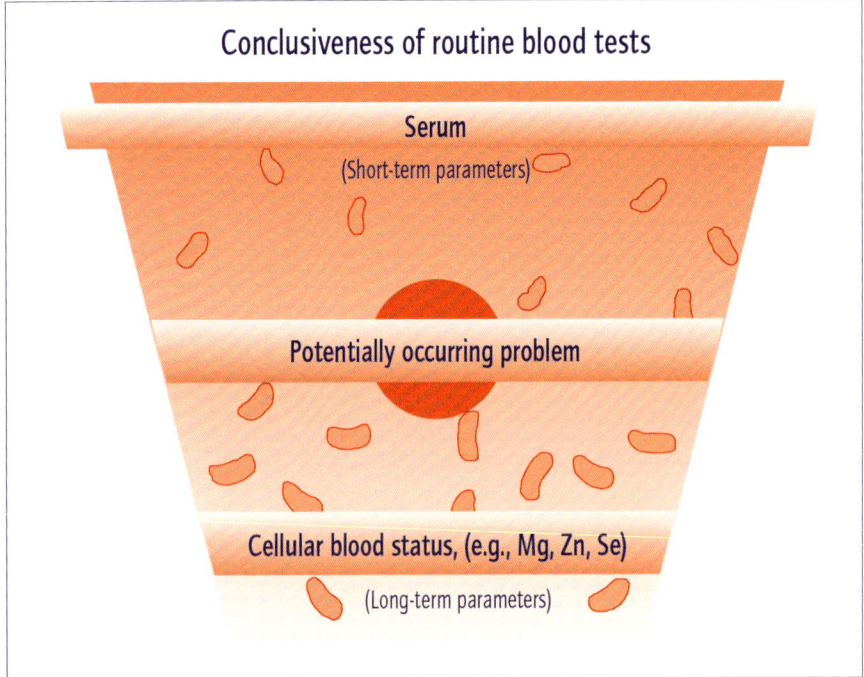

Fig. 33

Important information

- To conserve important micronutrients on the serum level, all of the body's own resources are mobilized, particularly at the cellular level. Therefore any deficiencies at the serum level are detected very late or not at all (see fig. 33).

- Optimization of the functional energy metabolism via a targeted intake of micronutrients ("Prescription for Energy") would not be possible without a cellular analysis (see chapters 1.3 and 1.4).

- **Important tip:** The intraerythrocytic analysis of micronutrients is optimal, because even in whole blood tests there are major fluctuations in measurements because of a short-term change in diet. We can see from among 36,760 case reports that the analyses of intraerythrocytic micronutrient concentrations are most conclusive as long-term parameters. Meanwhile various institutes offer whole blood analysis which conclusiveness is also limited for this reason (because 90% of magnesium is intraerythrocytic and not in whole blood). This should absolutely be taken into account.

3.4 CAUSES OF INCREASING DEFICIENCIES IN EXECUTIVES, TOP COMPETITIVE ATHLETES, AND IN ADULTS WITH ADHA

SALUTO was able to prove in many research projects and in a clinical study that even with a balanced diet the functional energy metabolism shows signs of biochemical disorders that are linked to impaired activity of certain enzymes, and thus lead to many disorders. At this point we will forgo a more detailed account of the findings.

A RESULT OF THE GREENHOUSE EFFECT

American biologists explain why we see an increasing deficiency in our cellular micronutrient balance in spite of a balanced diet: The effects of increasing CO_2 emissions on the reduction of micronutrient concentrations in today's food is not insignificant. The content and quantities of substances reported worldwide are outdated.

Today we must assume that a definite reduction of ingredients exists in our food. If losses of this magnitude were measured in only six months, then the actual losses over the past decades must be even bigger. This is said to be one of the main reasons why physically active people, in particular, are unable to attain an adequate micronutrient supply in spite of a balanced diet. In addition to the grave consequences of micronutrient losses due to the greenhouse effect shown in fig. 34, there are additional disturbing factors, such as incorrect preparation and storage-related losses.

Background knowledge

The American biologist Iraki Loladze of Princeton University in New Jersey already reported on initial tests in 2002, and found that the vastly increased CO_2 emissions over the past decades have resulted in a definite reduction of beneficial ingredients (see fig. 34). There is no other explanation for the results of our clinical study with 100 women and 76 students with a healthy diet. His research up to 2002 essentially describes two processes:

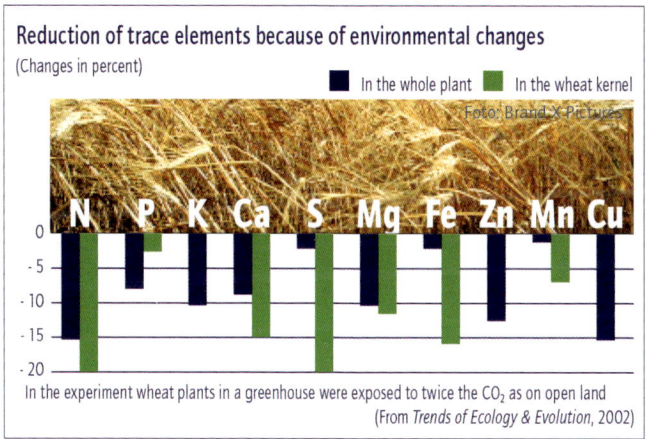

Fig. 34

1. The increased CO_2 emissions promote plant growth and thus crop yields, but at the expense of precious beneficial ingredients (trace elements, other micronutrients).
2. The higher CO_2 values limit the plants' evaporation of water; because less water evaporates from the leaves, less water is also absorbed from the ground. This diminished water balance leads to less availability of iron, magnesium, and zinc from the soil.

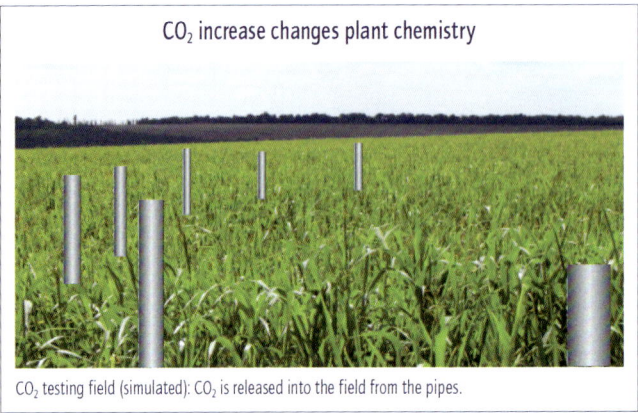

CO₂ testing field (simulated): CO₂ is released into the field from the pipes.

Fig. 35

The obvious conclusion is, we must assume that a decrease of beneficial ingredients in food exists today, but which scientists from various "lobbying" backgrounds continue to discount.

In a pilot project at the TU Braunschweig, Germany, scientists simulated the greenhouse effect in 2050 (see fig. 35). The results show a considerable decrease in micronutrients (zinc, selenium, as well as protein concentration) in the plants tested (with the exception of calcium).

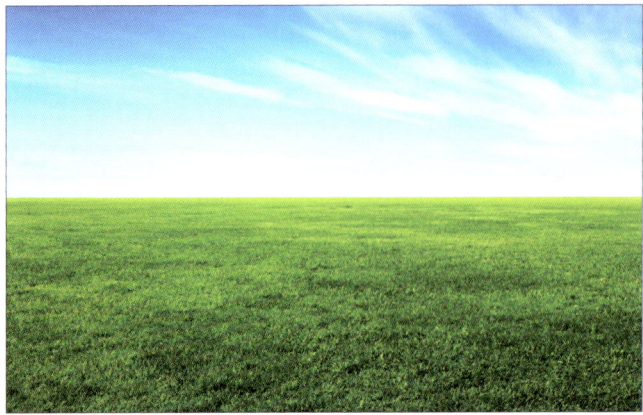

Plants will grow faster, but contain considerably fewer micronutrients. In the fall of 2008, a popular television program featured the results form the TU Braunschweig research in a testing field. In 2011, we measured the highest CO_2 emissions at 440 ppm. This was reported by the scientific institute Commonwealth Scientific and Industrial Research Organization (see fig. 36).

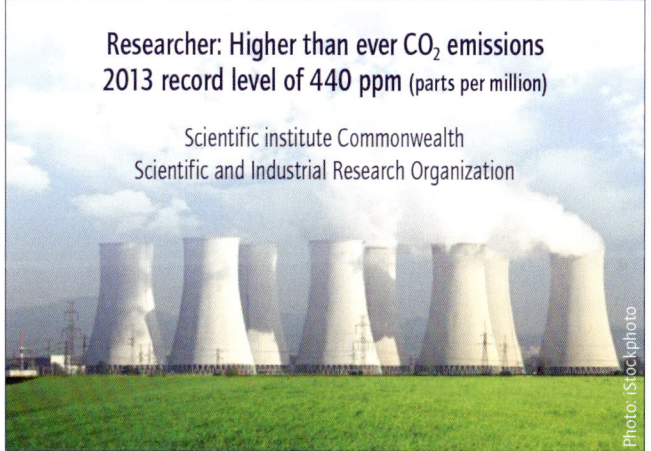

Fig. 36

An excerpt from an interview with Dr. Gerhard Rechkemmer, (President, Max Rubner Institue, Karlsruhe, Germany, German Federal Research Institute for Diet and Nutrition) and the author, published in *Alverde Magazine*, July 2013

Author: "There is evidence that the greenhouse effect can alter beneficial ingredients. A high CO_2 content makes plants grow tall but also absorb fewer minerals."

Dr. Rechkemmer: "That is correct! Our own growing experiments showed us that a high CO_2 content alters gluten in wheat with respect to the total amount and its composition. This in turn affects the flour's baking quality. Whether or not these changes are notable with respect to the German public's nutrition supply has to date not been characterized or researched."

A HEALTHY DIET: AN UNATTAINABLE OPTIMUM

Everyone is aware of the relationship between nutrition and performance capacity. Meanwhile, there are countless books that deal with this subject more or less objectively. We will therefore not offer any details here but rather focus on a good diet in general (for diet tips, see pg. 124) and on the qualitative and quantitative supplemental intake of micronutrients in particular, which are subject of a contentious debate between sports medicine and nutrition science specialists.

Only useful in combination

Based on the results we have shared so far, one could get the impression the executives and athletes depend on an additional targeted intake of micronutrients, and a good diet has much less of an impact on the micronutrient balance than previously thought.

But that is far from the truth. What is true is the absolute necessity of a personalized micronutrient formula (not based on a shotgun approach and the idea that "more is better"). But our many years of research show that only those who also have a balanced diet with lots of fruit and vegetables (and the many yet unexplored secondary nutrients they contain) can also absorb the additional micronutrients.

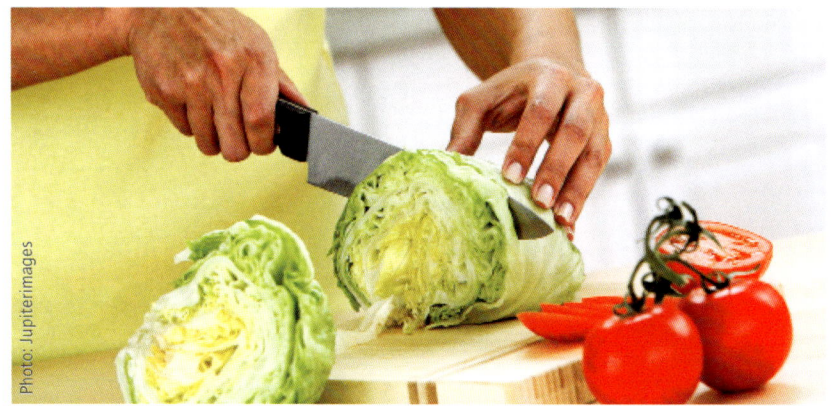

Fig. 37

Anyone who thinks he can ease his guilty conscience with a regular intake of vitamins, minerals, and trace elements—based on the motto "eat fast food and take pills"—did not understand the problem.

According to our research, the minimum requirement of eating approximately 600-800 g of fruit and vegetables per day (see fig. 37), was not attainable for the executives we tested and completely disregards the working world.

Of the 10,270 executives (entrepreneurs, executive managers, executive staff) we tested, 70% were dissatisfied with their dietary habits. More then 70% of these executives are physically active and yet still feel mentally and physically depleted. But they also talk about the enormous problem of maintaining a healthy diet while traveling, and attending meetings and business appointments. Even in top competitive athletes with good diets, the functional energy metabolism shows considerable impairments (see pg. 33, fig. 14), resulting in biochemical disorders of the functional energy metabolism and many health problems.

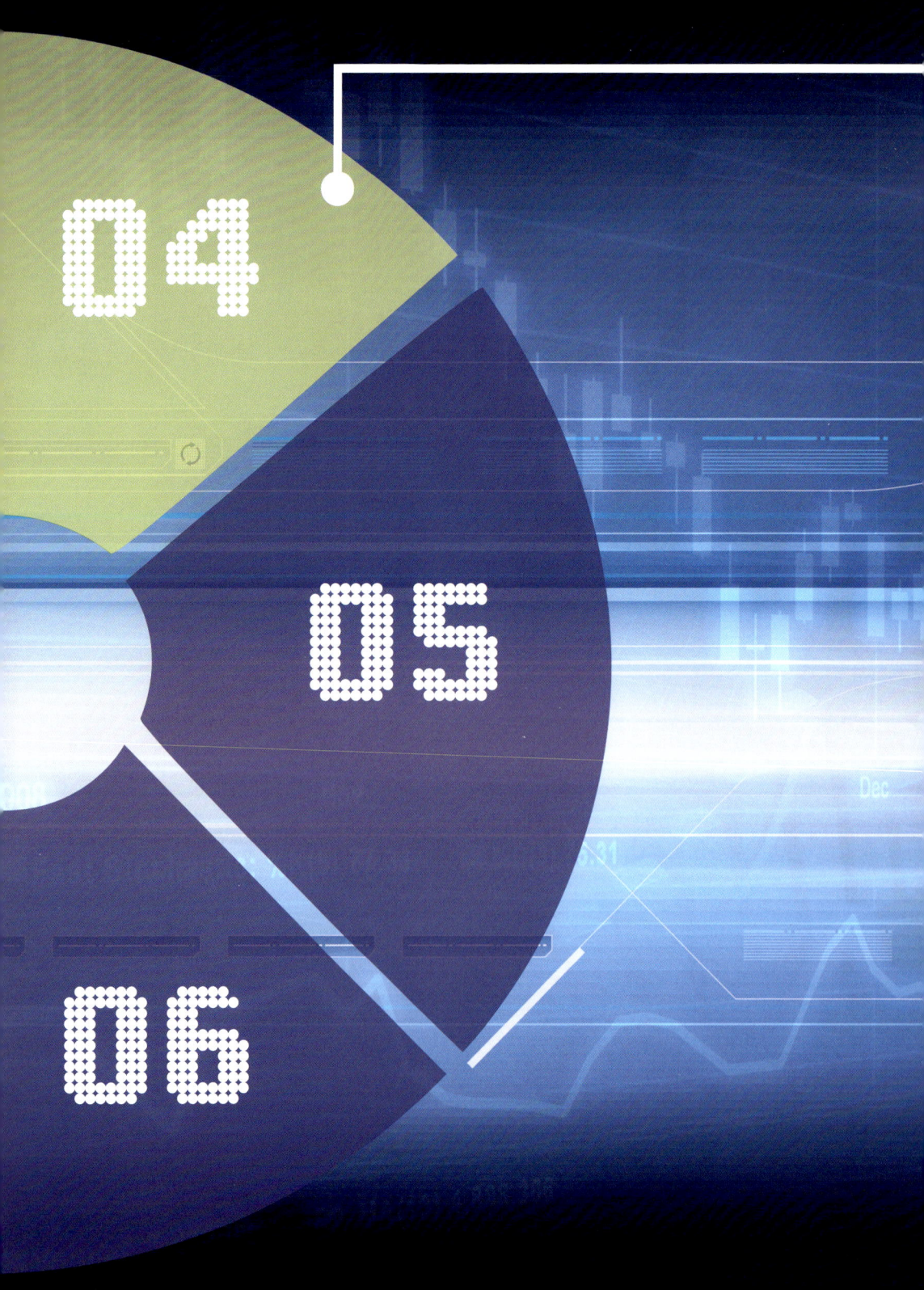

BIOCHEMISTRY OF HAPPINESS

4 BIOCHEMISTRY OF HAPPINESS

4.1 CONSEQUENCES OF BIOCHEMICAL DISORDERS

Typical ramifications of biochemical imbalances include insomnia, mental and physical performance fluctuations, and even to severe mood swings. Our extensive and comprehensive analyses of executives as well as top competitive athletes show a definite need for optimization in the area of brain-activating amino acids and some other basic micronutrients. Severe deficiencies that negatively affect the brain metabolism and sleep patterns, for example, the amino acids tryptophan, phenylalanine, and tyrosine (see fig. 38 and 40), were detected in 10,270 business executives and in top competitive athletes. Of the executives, 79% report increasing exhaustion and poor sleep quality.

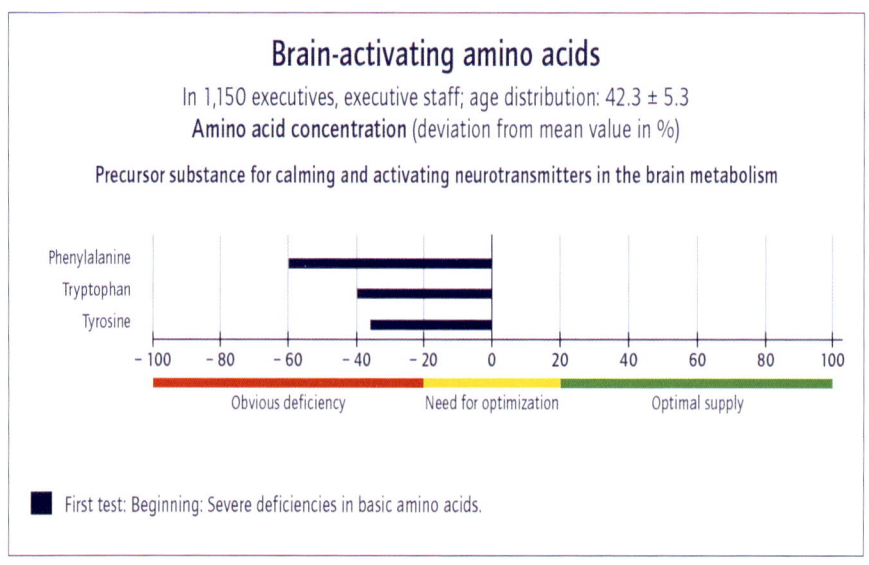

Fig. 38

Our results show their deviations from the average values (in %) of comparable people (age group, personal lifestyle, prior illnesses, exercise habits). At 20% above the mean values in amino acids, the executives and competitive athletes that were tested show no biochemical impairments in the functional energy metabolism (also see chapters 1.3 and 1.4).

Evaluation criteria for deviations from mean values:

- Up to -10% of the mean: slight deficiency
- Up to -20% of the mean: definite deficiency
- Up to -30% of the mean: blatant deficiency
- Up to +20% of the mean: optimization needed
- Up to > +21% of the mean: optimal supply

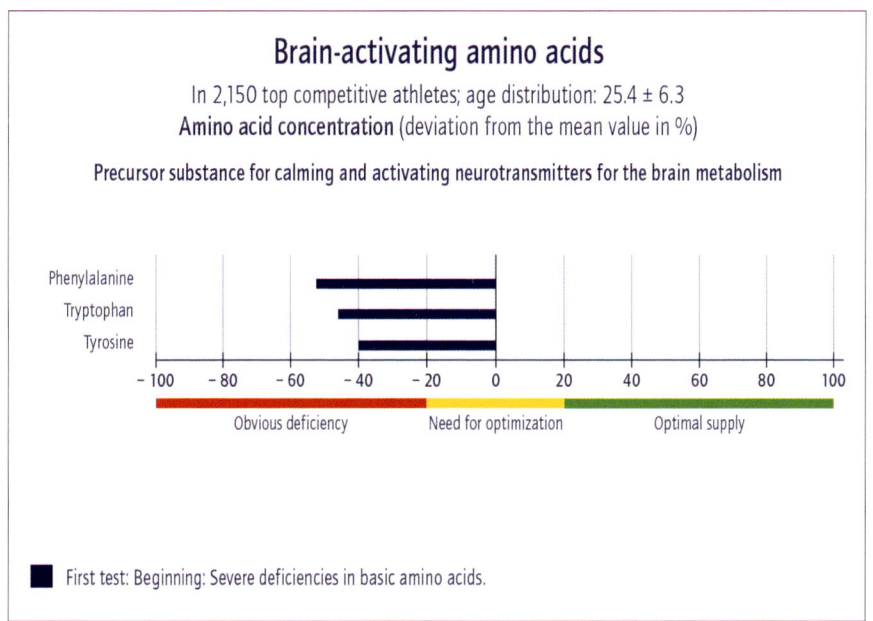

Fig. 39

These results show a definite deficiency in the supply of brain-activating amino acids. A lack of tryptophan verifiably results in poor sleep quality (fitful sleep). This in turn results in a definite decrease in mental alertness during the day. But also serotonin, which is fundamentally important to the moods of human beings, can no longer be adequately produced. The individual increasingly experiences chronic fatigue. It is extremely difficult to meet the tryptophan requirements, for instance, with a balanced diet.

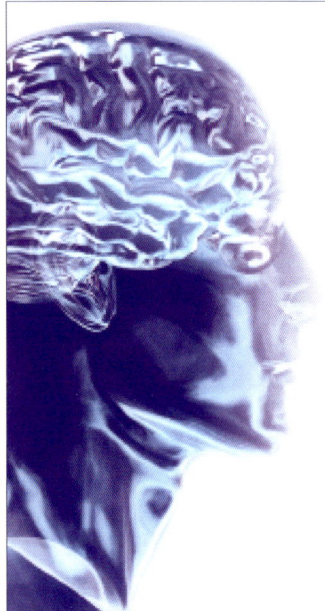

Mental performance capacity
With an optimal supply
of amino acids for the brain metabolism
(e.g., tryptophan)

Example:
Daily requirement of tryptophan: 3-6 mg/kg body weight
Competitive athlete: up to 7 mg/kg

Please note:
A cellular B_6 concentration that is too high
has an inhibiting effect;
effectiveness also depends on other
micronutrients, such as B-vitamins, Mg.

Fig. 40

Additional details on the functioning of individual amino acids can be found in chapter 4.3. We will further elaborate on the relationships there. Mental performance capacity verifiably also depends on an optimal supply of amino acids (tryptophan, phenylalanine, tyrosine). The daily requirements for tryptophan can be seen in fig. 40. Based on our experience from recent years, this number is between 3-6 mg/kg of body weight, for competitive athletes up to 7 mg/kg of body weight. Even with an optimal diet, it is extremely difficult to meet the requirement (see fig. 41).

BIOCHEMISTRY OF HAPPINESS

Even with an optimal nutrition, it is extremely difficult to meet the requirement (the example here is tryptophan).

Foods with high tryptophan content:

Food	Tryptophan content (mg/100g)
Nuts (e.g., cashews)	450
Cheese (Edam)	400
Wheat germ	330
Oats	186
Peas	100
Organic yoghurt	45
Meat/fish	approx. 200-250

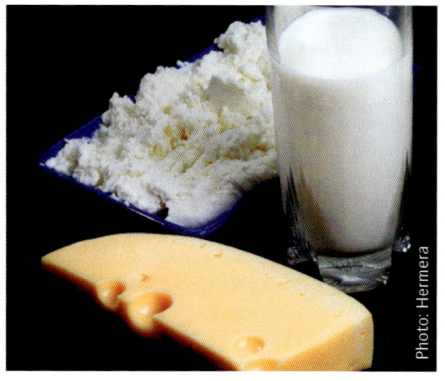

Photo: Hermera

Fig. 41

4.2 A LOOK AT THE INDIVIDUAL MEASUREMENTS

FUNCTIONAL ENERGY METABOLISM (METABOLITES AND ACIDS)

This measurement initially checks your energy metabolism function (see fig. 42). Our results show deviations from the mean values (in %) of comparable people (age group, personal lifestyle, prior illnesses, exercise habits). Where the dark blue bars meet the red bar, we can see the impairments in the activity of certain enzymes (accelerate chemical processes) that result in a verifiable decrease in energy production.

Lower metabolite concentrations are often due to an inadequate supply of carbon atoms that are transferred from amino acids to these intermediates of the citric acid cycle. The result is a decrease in energy production.

Brief digression on the functional energy metabolism

The citric acid cycle is the central switch point of the entire metabolism. Here are the breakdown paths of carbohydrates, fats, and proteins. A deficiency in basic micronutrients (amino acids, vitamins, minerals, trace elements) results in an impairment of the power stations of the cells (mitochondrial dysfunction). Different metabolic products are measured here. An increase or decrease of measured substances indicate certain impairments of the energy metabolism and are associated with a decrease in energy production.

Different acids and metabolites are measured in the citric acid cycle (e.g., citric acid, cis-aconitic acid, alpha-ketoglutaric acid, succinic acid, fumaric acid, malic acid, pyruvate) that, based on our results, point to impaired activity of important enzymes in the energy metabolism (see fig. 42).

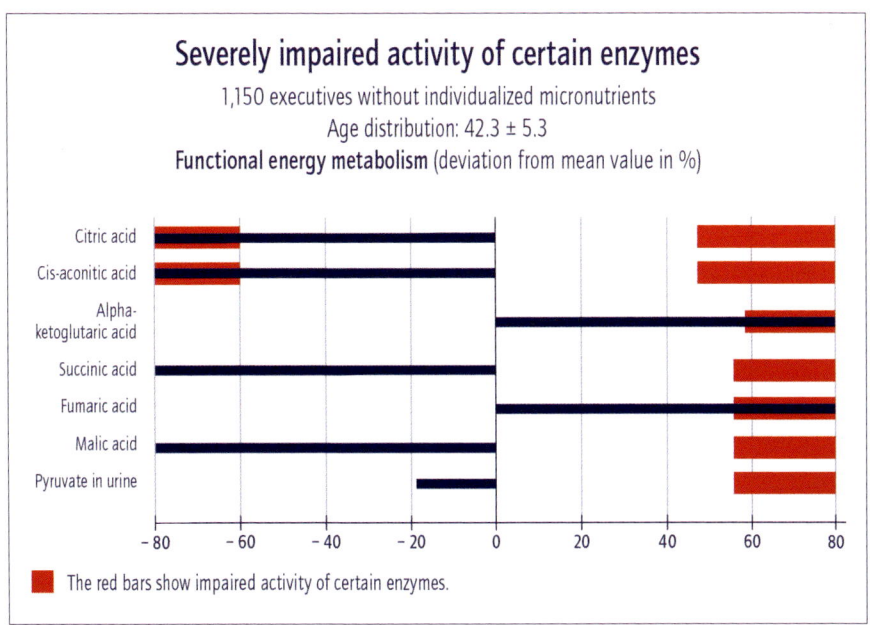

Fig. 42

INTERPRETATION OF THE FUNCTIONAL ENERGY METABOLISM PARAMETERS

Citric acid

< -60% or > +60% of mean value indicates for micronutrient deficiencies (enzymatic inhibition).

Cis-aconitic acid

< -60% or > +60% of mean value show impaired activity of certain enzymes.

Alpha-ketoglutaric acid

+60% above the mean value shows mitochondrial dysfunction as well as impaired breakdown of some basic amino acids.

Succinic acid

+60% of mean value signals B_2 and coenzyme Q_{10} deficiency—key function in the mitochondria.

Fumaric acid

+30% of mean value signals B_2 and coenzyme Q_{10} deficiency—key function in the mitochondria.

Malic acid

+30% of mean value. All three citric acid cycle metabolites, succinic, fumaric, and malic acid signal a vitamin B deficiency: An increase in these metabolites can lead to an interruption in the electron transport, and thus decreased energy production.

Pyruvate

+40% of mean value indicates impaired function of the pyruvate dehydrogenese because of a possible vitamin B deficiency.

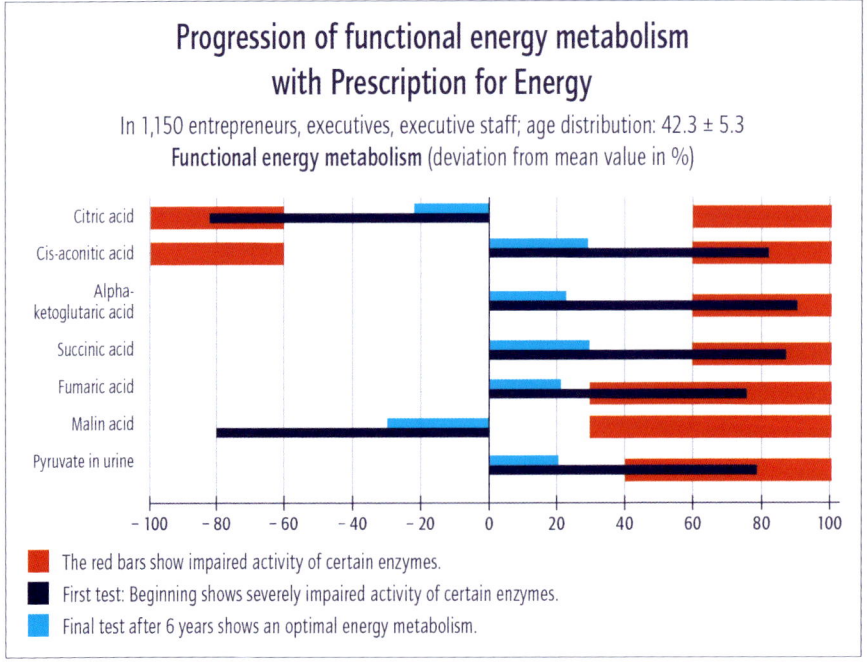

Fig. 43

Urine tests done over an extended period of time on executives and top athletes show a definite impact of the individualized micronutrient prescriptions on the functional energy metabolism. A normalization or economization of the metabolism can be achieved with an individualized Prescription for Energy.

Fig. 44 shows the progression of the functional energy metabolism in 1,150 executives at the beginning of and after five years (final test). Semi-annual checkups during the evaluation period resulted in an adjustment to the micronutrient prescription (fig. 16, pg. 36, shows the functional energy metabolism of 2,150 top competitive athletes).

SPECIAL INTRACELLULAR MICRONUTRIENT ANALYSES

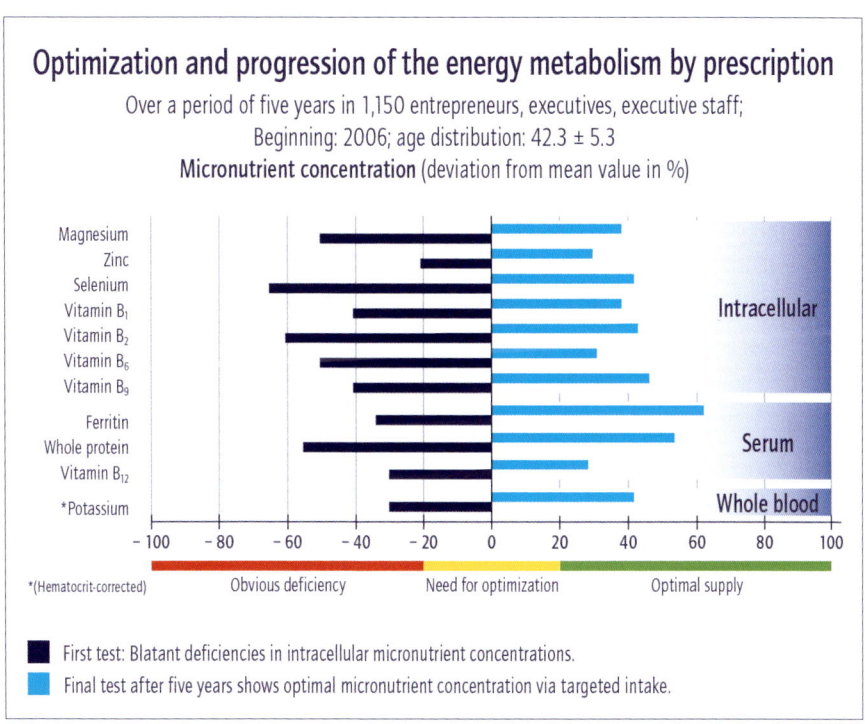

Fig. 44

Correct energy and micronutrient diagnostics are the alpha and omega (see pg. 65). A routine blood test ascertains vitamins, minerals, and trace elements in blood serum, but not in the blood cells. The concentration of many trace elements and minerals is predominately cellular (present in the red blood cells). This is also true for vitamins B_1, B_2, B_6, and B_9. Blood serum tests are not conclusive with respect to the actual supply of micronutrients to the blood cells.

Few institutes in Germany conduct these tests. Evaluation is based on an extensive data bank of 10,270 executives, 11,150 top competitive athletes, and 15,340 previously physically inactive people.

Our results show the deviations from mean values (in %) of comparable people (age group, personal lifestyle, prior illnesses, exercise habits). Fig. 44 shows the optimization and progression of the energy metabolism by prescription in 1,150 executives, at the beginning of and after five years. The individualized micronutrient formulas are continually adjusted based on current facts and conditions via two semi-annual checkups.

Biochemical disorders that resulted in impaired activity of certain enzymes, particularly in the functional energy metabolism, are triggered by the various micronutrient deficiencies. Targeted replenishment of micronutrients verifiably leads to a normalization of the energy metabolism and a decrease in disorders.

With respect to the executives, as well as the top athletes, were the very low cellular B-vitamin concentrations. The folic acid concentration, in particular, supports the brain metabolism. Our results show that people who are under a lot of professional stress as well as competitive athletes have considerable deficiencies in the cellular folic acid concentration and have an increased tendency to mental fatigue.

AMINO ACID MEASUREMENT AND ITS DIFFERENTIATON

Amino acids as nutrients have a direct impact on your personal well-being. By choosing the right foods you can influence your status and achieve a good mood. A more detailed description of the functionality of individual amino acids and their importance to the brain and nutrient metabolism can be found in chapter 4.3.

From the comprehensive long-term analyses, we have been able to ascertain mean values for each group of people (executives, top competitive athletes, and physically inactive people). A group-specific deviation above 25% of these mean values indicates an optimal supply of the specific amino acids.

When measuring we differentiate amino acids that
- are significant to the preservation of the function of various connective tissue structures (tendons, ligaments, muscles, cartilage) and the immune system, such as arginine, methionine, proline, and glutamine;
- are important to the optimization of the energy metabolism and for neurotransmitter activity, such as alanine, aspartic acid, and tyrosine;
- are important to the stabilization of the energy metabolism, such as BCAAs (leucine, isoleucine, valine); and
- have an effect on the brain metabolism as a precursor substance for calming or activating neurotransmitters.

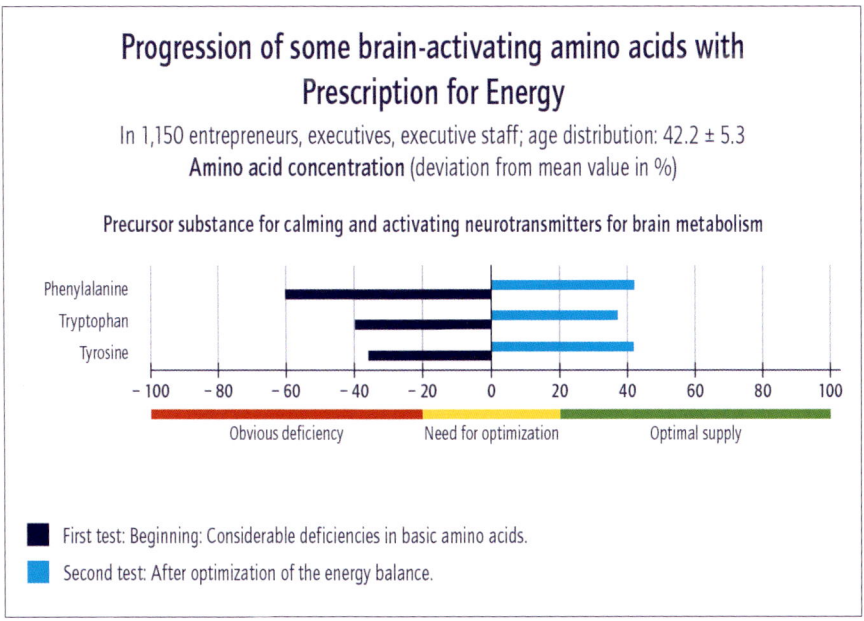

Fig. 45

Groups of people who are at > 25% of the respective ascertained mean value show psychophysical stability, no exhaustion, and feel even-tempered and able to withstand stress. This is true for executives, top competitive athletes, as well as people with

ADHD. Groups of people who are at < 20% of the respective ascertained mean values show increasing disorders (e.g., poor sleep quality, agitation, not being able to unwind after work).

Fig. 45. offers another explicit view of what the initial supply of brain-activating amino acids (phenylalanine, tryptophan, tyrosine) looked like in 1,150 executives. The targeted intake of amino acids they lacked verifiably resulted in improved sleep quality and a considerably improved overall mood. The same effects are seen in the 2,150 top competitive athletes (see chapter 1.4).

In top competitive athletes, the amino acids that are fundamentally important to the preservation of function and stabilization of connective tissue structures (ligaments, tendons, muscles, cartilage) show no injuries in the non-contact (i.e., without outside influence) area at values above 25% of the mean (see fig. 47).

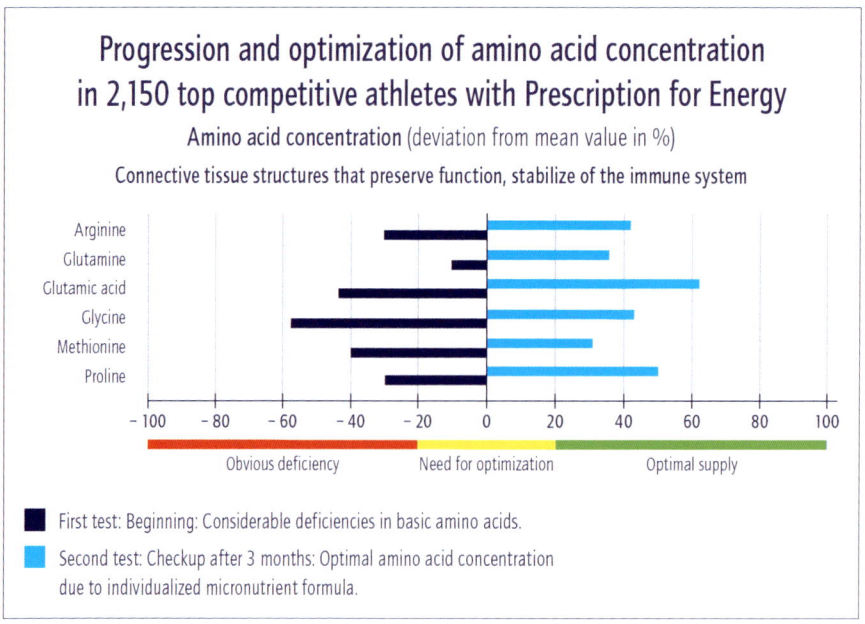

Fig. 46

DEMAND ON THE BODY'S OWN STRUCTURAL PROTEINS IN THE ENERGY METABOLISM

Newly developed parameters, called *pyridinium crosslinks*, can show early deficiencies in the energy metabolism (i.e., demand on the body's own structural proteins). Taking this measurement during the stress phase (regeneration, intense training, and competition phase) is recommended, especially for top competitive athletes.

Our bones are subject to constant buildup and breakdown. Bone buildup predominates until about the age of 30, which coincides with a continuous increase in bone density. After that the course changes in direction of bone breakdown, and at some point the breakdown outweighs the buildup process.

Longer lasting bone breakdown processes lead to a decrease in bone density and finally osteoporosis with a higher risk of bone fractures. The bones and also the cartilage consists of collagen molecules that are stabilized via crosslinking. In bone these crosslinks are primarily *deoxypyridinolin (DPD)*; in cartilage however, it is *pyridinoline (PD)*. During increased breakdown processes, these crosslinks are released into the blood and then excreted in the urine. The amount of excreted pyridinium crosslinks depends on the extent of the breakdown processes. Since neither the newly synthesized bone substance nor the collagen-containing nutritional components impact the excretions, *deoxypyridinolin* is, at this time, considered to be the best marker for selective assessment of bone resorption.

Based on our experience, this parameter is a good indicator for measuring pyridinium crosslinks in top competitive athletes to determine the extent the athletes' energy metabolism has stressed the body's own structural proteins that are fundamentally important to preserving the function of connective tissue structures (ligaments, tendon, cartilage).

Elevated PD and DPD values can show to what extent the most intense athletic demands stress the cartilage and bone metabolism.

In many athletes, definite micronutrient deficiencies are detected that verifiably inhibit many enzymes during energy production and thereby quickly cause the organism to draw on the body's own structural proteins. Since neither PD nor DPD is ingested with food, the assignation of crosslinks in the urine can take place independently from the current nutritional status. The ratio of PD: DPD gives more detailed information about the breakdown location.

If top competitive athletes do not receive an individualized micronutrient formula, energy demand is placed on the body's own structural proteins (arginine, methionine, proline) which are then verifiably no longer available for preserving the function of stressed connective tissue structures (see chapter 1.4). A targeted, individualized formula reduces the demand on the body's own structural proteins after just a few months (see fig. 47), and this provides optimal injury protection.

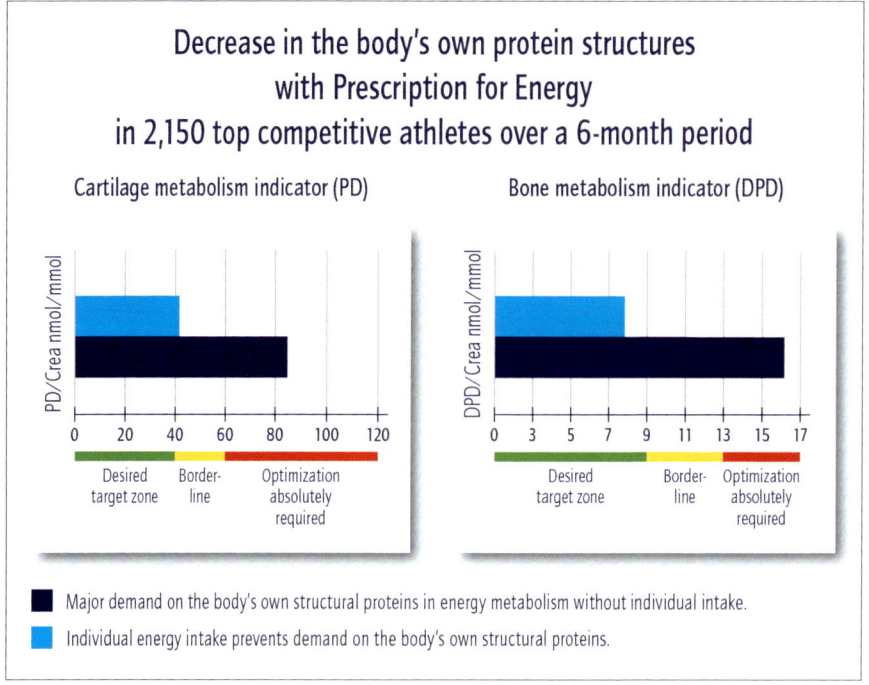

Fig. 47

COMPREHENSIVE WORLDWIDE DATA BANK (36,760 PEOPLE)

The comprehensive analyses of the individual parameters can only lead to practical action with the appropriate formula if the different groups of people (executives, entrepreneurs, executive staff, recreational and top competitive athletes, physically inactive people, and people with different prior illnesses) are taken into account. The individualized formulas are developed based on comparable data from the respective group of people and the respective deviations from the mean values.

We did not find any biochemical impairments in the individual groups of people above 25% of the respective mean values of the functional energy metabolism. Many disorders (such as increasing exhaustion, poor sleep quality, agitation) are directly linked to an adequate energy and micronutrient intake.

Important advice

An evaluation of the comprehensive analyses must always be done in relation to the group of people, age, sex, prior illnesses, and type of job. With top competitive athletes, the type of sport and the timing of respective training and competition phases are crucial.

4.3 THE ROLE OF MICRONUTRIENTS: HOW MICRONUTRIENTS REALLY HELP

Here we pick only a few micronutrients as examples and forgo more detailed biochemical explanations.

GENERAL ASPECTS OF AMINO ACIDS

An optimal supply of amino acids ensures performance capacity and injury protection. Proteins are basic building blocks of all the body's cells and control all biochemical processes in the body. As basic building blocks for muscle fiber and as structural protein and protective protein of the cartilage substance, bones, tendons, and skin, proteins are the body's most important structural elements.

Inside the organism a constant protein buildup and breakdown takes place. Amino acids are the basic building blocks of proteins. Our amino acid storage is small, only about 120 g, located in the blood plasma and mostly in the muscles and cellular structures. A daily high-quality protein supply from food is advisable since the organism is unable to sufficiently store amino acids.

Essential and non-essential amino acids

The human body is unable to produce 8 of the 22 amino acids. These essential amino acids must be supplied from food. Meanwhile, some semi-essential amino acids have also been identified whose regular supply is necessary to take on some important tasks in the metabolism.

However, to what extent the typical classifications as essential and non-essential amino acids will be retained in the future is questionable because some research has shown that the boundaries between these two groups can be fluid at times. We have been able to show that even non-essential amino acids can be essential in certain situations. At present, 9 of the 20 amino acids (essential) are by definition irreplaceable for humans, and these are:

- Histidine
- Valine
- Leucine
- Isoleucine
- Lysine
- Methionine
- Phenylalanine
- Threonine
- Tryptophan

Conditionally essential amino acids include:
- Arginine
- Glycine
- Cysteine
- Glutamine
- Tyrosine
- Serine
- Taurine

Non-essential, but still important, amino acids are:
- Alanine
- Aspartic acid
- Asparagine
- Glutamic acid
- Ornithine
- Proline

Tasks and functions of several amino acids

In natural proteins, amino acids are always present in an L-shape. The L specifies the spatial structure of the molecule. Aside from a few exceptions, the body can only use L-amino acids. So if here we refer to amino acids, we always mean L-amino acids (e.g., glutamine = L-glutamine).

High-quality amino acids carry out important tasks in the organism:

- During energy metabolism: synthesis from creatine phosphate; build up glycogen stores; support burning of fatty acids;
- Improved mental and muscle regeneration;
- Optimal protection from injury and immune stabilization;
- Optimal buildup of bradytrophic tissue structures.

Amino acids—guarantor for mental and cognitive performance capacity

Mental and physical performance capacity is no coincidence. A good mood, great performance, and creativity all depends on an adequate supply of amino acids that impact the functional energy metabolism. Mental and physical stress can significantly increase the demand.

Amino acids as nutrients have a direct impact on your personal well-being. With the right selection of foods, you can have a direct effect on your status and achieve a good mood. Euphoria and optimism are mirror images of your amino acids. With an optimal supply of the listed basic amino acids, misery and anxiety will quickly fade away.

Protein—quality instead of quantity

Our body requires sufficient protein to build up and maintain its musculature. To date, a daily requirement of between 1.0 and 1.8 g per kg of body weight was deemed appropriate. From today's perspective this is not worth discussing. To maintain muscle it is not the overall quantity of protein that is important but the quality, for example collagen peptide (arginine, methionine, proline), to preserve function of the various connective tissue structures and the brain-activating amino acids.

Animal protein (e.g., ocean fish, lean meat, eggs) is of particularly high quality. A combination of different food proteins, such as potatoes with eggs, is optimal. When consuming fats, plant fats (e.g., olive oil, rapeseed oil) with high amounts of unsaturated fatty acids are best. The general rule applies that eating several small portions is better than consuming three large meals, especially for athletes. It is best to spread meals out to six to eight small portions over the course of the day.

IMPORTANT FOR THE BRAIN METABOLISM

The comprehensive analyses in 21,420 executives top competitive athletes as well as 15,340 previously physically inactive people show definite optimization potential. Meanwhile the everyday stresses increasingly lead to exhaustion and sometimes even burnout. The battery is empty on all levels. There is a pervasive feeling of "I can't do this anymore", and "I feel powerless, unmotivated, and sad."

Amino acids, such as phenylalanine, tryptophan, and tyrosine, are particularly important to the brain metabolism. All of the people who describe these symptoms are at 20% below our mean values. We describe the link between, for instance, mental performance capacity and the amino acid tryptophan (see pg. 80). When we look at the entire energy balance of 4,150 executives (see chapter 1.3) with an age distribution of 44.3 ± 9.2, it becomes obvious that next to a few other micronutrients the listed amino acids are present in particularly low concentrations. After a targeted micronutrient therapy, especially the intake of amino acids, many biochemical impairments of the functional energy metabolism have been remedied (see pg. 164, fig. 89).

Phenylalanine—a mood-brightener

Phenylalanine is a precursor to the catecholamines dopamine, adrenaline, and noradrenaline. Impairments of the catecholamine metabolism are involved in the emergence of increasing exhaustion. L-phenylalanine has a mood and concentration-influencing property. All of the people tested who complained about increasing exhaustion showed considerable deficiencies in this amino acid.

Tryptophan—the amino acid that helps you sleep

Tryptophan is a precursor to the neurotransmitters serotonin and the hormone melatonin. A serotonin deficiency is being debated as a significant factor in sleep disturbances and depressive moodiness. Balancing a serotonin deficiency can be achieved with an additional tryptophan intake. Unlike serotonin, tryptophan can overcome the blood-brain barrier and reach the brain. There it is transformed into serotonin.

As previously mentioned, it is extremely difficult to meet tryptophan requirements through a balanced diet (see fig. 41, pg. 83). Based on our experiences in recent years, executives require 5 mg/kg body weight. Top Competitive athletes verifiably require 6-7 mg/kg body weight. These deficiencies gradually increase over time, and the affected person feels increasingly exhausted, sleeps badly, and has mood swings. The arbitrary intake of tryptophan at night before bed is absolutely not recommended. This should only be done after appropriate diagnostics (see pg. 82). Intake of tryptophan is counterproductive with the use of antidepressants and existing bronchial asthma.

Tryptophan is used regularly and successfully for insomnia and increasing mood fluctuations. For a therapeutic effect, raising the serotonin and melatonin levels in the brain is of obvious importance. For insomnia dosages of 250, up to 1,000 mg/d are recommended depending on blood test results.

Important advice

Tryptophan resorption is slow. It should be taken approximately two hours prior to bedtime. It takes approximately four to five days for a noticeable effect with increasing therapy duration. It is suitable for chronic insomnia and can also be used for withdrawal in cases of sleeping pill dependency. In some cases, additional blood tests may be necessary for tryptophan diagnostics in order to get a more conclusive result for the individual (see fig. 48).

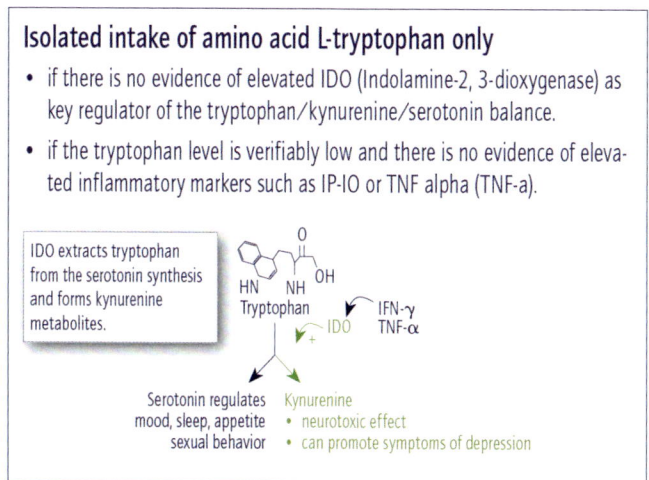

Fig. 48

AMINO ACIDS—THE ENGINE FOR BODY TISSUE AND FUNCTION

Preserving the body's own reserves

Recent research results show that amino acid consumption for the body's own carbohydrate production (gluconeogenesis) is significantly greater than previously thought.

Preservation of the amino acid allocation can be achieved with:

- good basic endurance and a subsequently well-trained fat metabolism,
- carbohydrate intake (40-60 g per hour of exertion), and
- amino acid supply (10-15 g per hour of exertion).

If the athlete has good basic endurance and consumes an adequate amount of carbohydrates during exertion, he is better able to preserve amino acids. But if there is a lack of amino acid and carbohydrate intake during intense or long training units, the amino acid reserves in the musculature and blood drop significantly. This results in an insufficient supply of amino acids to build up muscles, tendons, and ligaments, as well as the immune system, thereby considerably increasing the risk of injury. The elasticity of, for instance, the ligament apparatus decreases significantly because no sufficient quantities of amino acids (arginine, methionine, proline) are available to preserve function (see fig. 21, pg. 48).

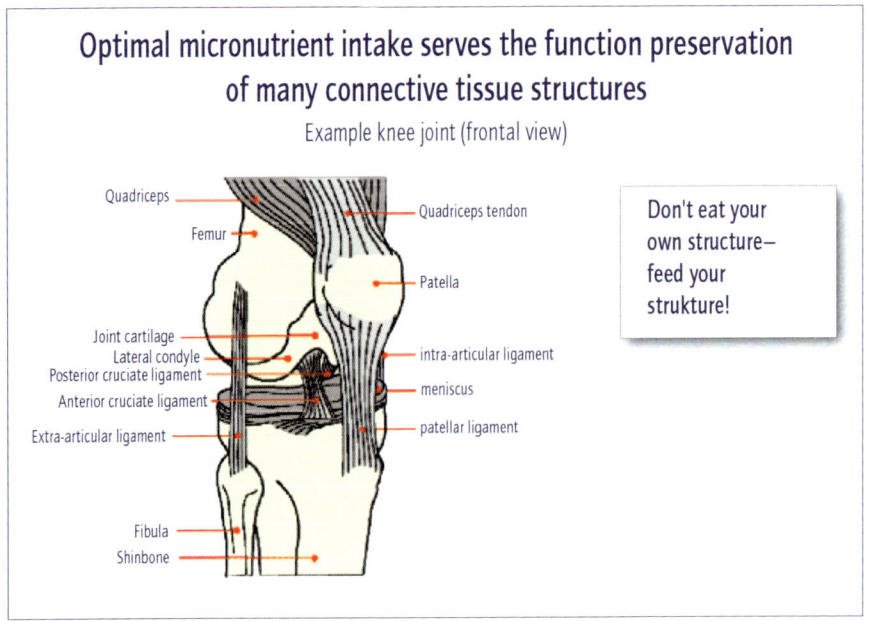

Fig. 49

Amino acids protect connective tissue structures during major stress

Because every organ is surrounded by connective tissue, a healthy connective tissue represents an optimal prerequisite for efficient, productive organ performance. An adults' connective tissue weighs approximately 13 kg and interconnects the organs and the nerves. Connective tissue structures also connect muscles to bone.

But who isn't familiar with this dilemma: Many performance-oriented recreational athletes experience increasing discomfort in the Achilles tendon, the hip, and the knee. These may be initial symptoms of poorly-formed connective tissue structures that become vulnerable under major stress. Vulnerable connective tissues that are particularly affected are:

- joint cartilage,
- ligaments and tendons,
- joint capsules and
- intervertebral discs.

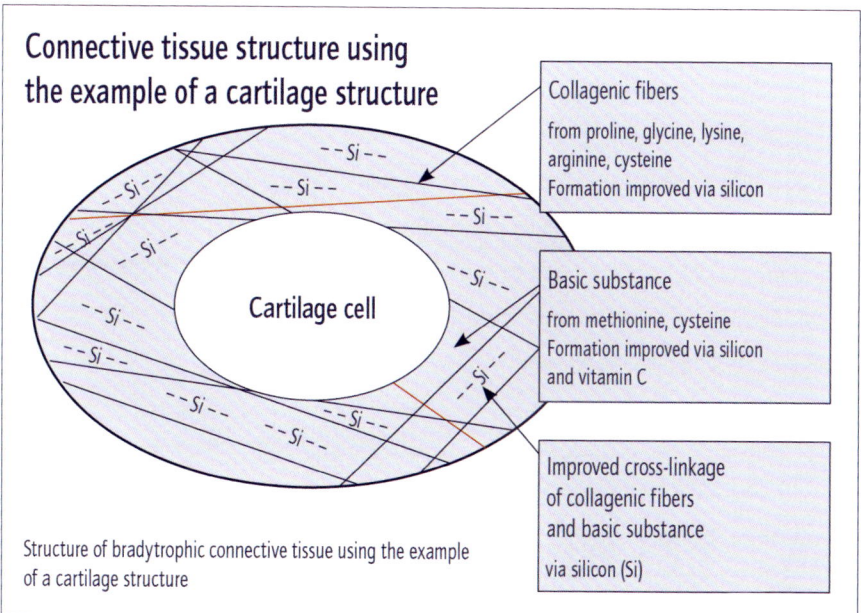

Fig. 50

Beginning, early complaints do not have to happen! An optimal diet and a targeted intake of amino acids can vitally strengthen your connective tissue. Our research in recreational as well as professional athletes has shown that fundamental deficiencies in bradytrophic, tissue-building amino acids (proline, glycine, lysine, arginine, methionine, and cysteine) exist specifically with these types of medical problems. With a targeted change in diet that includes more siliceous foods and the necessary supplemental intake of a high-quality amino acid blend many minor physical complaints can be avoided before they happen (see pg. 33, fig. 14, pg. 34, fig. 15).

THE OMEGA-3 INDEX: MEASURE FOR A GOOD MOOD (SEROTONIN METABOLISM)

Today the biochemical significance of omega fatty acids to the preservation of basic functional sequences in our metabolism is undisputed. The most important omega-3 fatty acids include:

- Alpha linoleic acid (simplest fatty acid)
- Eicosapentaenoic acid (EPA)
- Docosahexaenoic acid (DHA)

Alpha linoleic acid, the most basic fatty acid in the omega-3 fatty acid metabolism can be found in ferns, mosses, and some plant-based oils like linseed and rapeseed oil. The human organism can barely transform shorter-chain alpha linoleic acid (about 5-10%) into EPA and DHA. For this reason, the health-promoting effects of EPA and DHA cannot be gleaned from the intake of plant-based alpha linoleic acid. The following foods contain omega-3 fatty acids:

Omega-3 fatty acid content per 100 g	
Linseed oil	54.2 g
Rapeseed oil	9.2 g
Herring	2.3 g
Salmon	0.65 g
Mackerel	0.95 g

EPA and DHA are indispensible components of every cell membrane and thus essential to good health. They

- strengthen the immune system
- have an anti-inflammatory effect
- support the oxygen supply to organs
- lower-elevated blood fat and
- increase concentration and mental performance capacity

Now there is a omega-3 index, which is an indicator for serotonin production in the brain metabolism. When the percentual share of these two omega-3 fatty acids (EPA, DHA) in the erythrocytes is too low in EPA and DHA and the omega-3 index is < 8%, it is likely that mood fluctuations will increase considerably. In top competitive athletes, an omega-3 index of > 8% can verifiably have an anti-inflammatory effect after intense training and competition phases and offer good protection from muscle injuries. A therapeutic effect in cases of increasing exhaustion can be achieved with concentrations of at least 840 mg EPA and 560 mg DHA.

MAGNESIUM: MULTI-TALENT AMONG MINERALS

Magnesium takes part in more than 300 enzymatic processes. These are directly linked to the energy storage substance ATP (adenosine triphosphate). Magnesium plays a critical role in muscle contraction, stimulus conduction in nerve and muscle cells, stabilization of cell membranes, and the regulation of heart muscle function. An adequate supply increases stress tolerance and guards against premature exhaustion of cellular energy deposits and electrolytes. A magnesium deficiency increases potassium permeability, which impairs cellular potassium replenishment and negatively affects physical performance capacity and heart rate. Its antagonistic effect towards calcium protects the heart muscle cell from calcium overload. Thus magnesium economizes the heart muscle's bioenergetics, particularly during high stress, and prevents cardiac arrhythmia.

Typical symptoms of a magnesium deficiency can be:

- Keeping composure during stress phases and problems
- Muscle weakness
- Agitation
- Tendency for painful muscle and calf cramps
- Poor sleep quality and verifiably worsening regeneration and training adaptation

The results from our clinical study show that the magnesium serum concentration significantly increases statistically while the cellular concentration diminishes.

Conclusion: The magnesium balance status quo can only be ascertained via special cellular blood tests. More than 85% of the executives we tested have definite deficiencies in the cellular magnesium concentration and sleep fitfully at night.

Better stress tolerance for executives

The group of executives with cellular magnesium deficiencies shows considerably higher cortisol values during stress phases and has trouble unwinding after work and sleeping at night. The targeted intake of magnesium resulted in improved stress tolerance and sleeping patterns. In people with borderline thyroid hormones tending to hyperthyroidism (see fig. 27, pg. 56), a targeted intake can significantly reduce an increasing strain on the vegetative nervous system (sympathicotonia).

No optimal endurance without magnesium

Loss of intracellular magnesium in particular can lead to performance loss. About 80% of cellular ATP forms a complex bond with magnesium. Magnesium loses its binding partner during stress-related ATP consumption. This results in an intracellular release of magnesium and losses in the tissues. Because of the shift from intra- to extracellular space, the magnesium levels can temporarily be deceptively high, even though a deficiency exists. The kidneys react to the high magnesium level with increased excretion and thereby promote magnesium depletion.

An optimal cellular magnesium concentration is 25% above mean values of (55 mg/l ery), but can only be ascertained with special diagnostics. Cellular deficiencies require long-term intake of magnesium. Short-term intake for four to six weeks cannot replenish the cellular stores.

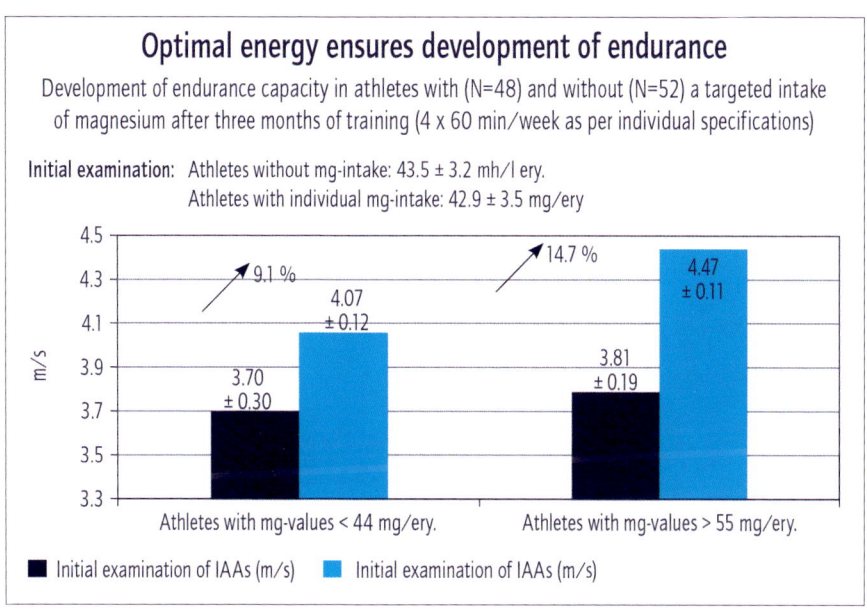

Fig. 51

In many of the studies we performed we were able to see a direct link to an optimal cellular magnesium concentration. During a three month training phase, 48 athletes did not receive any magnesium supplements while the other group of 52 athletes took a chewable magnesium supplement of 35 mg, with breakfast, lunch, and dinner (dosage based on measured magnesium concentration). Ferritin levels in both groups of athletes showed an adequate iron supply with 80.9 ± 8.9. Measured against the fixed threshold, the endurance capacity of athletes with a higher cellular magnesium concentration < 44 mg/l ery. developed by 4 mmol/l, only 9.1% (from 3.70 m/s ± 0.30 to 4.07 m/s ± 0.12), while the athletes with a magnesium concentration of > 55 mg/l ery. were able to develop the fixed threshold by 14.7% (from 3.81 m/s ± 0.19 to 4.47 m/s ± 0.11) (see fig. 51). Training volume was the same for both groups.

The significance of these parameters for the development of endurance capacity is particularly evident here.

Analogous to this study, the Gießen triathlon study from 1994 (Geiss et al.) produced similar results. In a double blind, randomized test, 23 athletes were given either magnesium or a placebo over a period of three months. The group with the targeted magnesium intake was able to increase their performance capacity by an average 12%.

Tips for a magnesium-rich diet

- Mineral water with magnesium content higher than 100 mg/l is recommended. Drink plenty of water!

- A common mistake: taking magnesium right before competing. This can be very stressful to the gastrointestinal system. For this reason we recommend regular intake after a competition.

- Avoid magnesium intake during athletic exertion. Muscle cramps during athletic competitions are usually not caused by a magnesium deficiency but are the result of insufficient preparatory training and a stress-induced sodium deficiency.

OPTIMAL IRON SUPPLY: ENSURES PERFORMANCE CAPACITY

As a basic building block of the red blood pigment hemoglobin, iron is essential to the transport of oxygen in the blood and the oxygen supply for the cellular energy metabolism (in the mitochondria = power stations of the cells). A good iron supply is vital to an optimal mental and physical performance capacity and for immune system function. Without oxygen, our muscle cells are unable to produce energy. Iron deficiency is the most often diagnosed mineral deficiency in sports medicine. The athlete feels tired and run down, and doesn't regenerate sufficiently after intense training.

Symptoms of an iron deficiency can be:

- diminished performance capacity,
- overall fatigue,
- anemia,
- lacerations at the corners of the mouth, and
- impaired hair and nail growth.

Because of the higher loss of iron via the gastrointestinal tract, with sweat and urine, athletes have higher iron requirements that are not always met by a balanced diet that includes meat. Next to athletes with a vegetarian diet, female endurance athletes as well as adolescent male and female athletes due to menstruation and physical growth, have a higher risk of developing an iron deficiency. Long-distance runners in particular suffer from iron deficiencies, primarily via perspiration (0.3-0.7 mg/l) and stress-induced blood loss in the gastrointestinal tract (1 ml blood contains 0.5 mg iron).

Ascertaining the iron status

Measuring iron in serum is not suitable for diagnosing an iron deficiency. Because the ferritin level in serum correlates well with tissue iron, this test is considered standard. An iron deficiency exists at 1 µg/l serum ferritin (equivalent to approximately 8-10 mg stored iron). For athletes, regular ferritin assessments are absolutely essential. But physically active executives often show signs of ferritin deficiencies. In women, serum ferritin values of < 40 are already associated with diffuse hair loss. In endurance athletes, ferritin values should be in the following ranges in order to achieve an optimal development of their endurance capacity:

Physically active women > 60 µg/ml
Physically active men > 120 µg/ml.

There are ongoing divisive discussions regarding the level of optimal ferritin values. Based on our experiences with 11,150 athletes and completed studies, we have been able to ascertain the following reference data. Our test results show the importance of an optimal iron supply for the development of endurance capacity. The already low starting ferritin levels in athletes who did not receive a targeted iron intake dropped even after the three month training phase. These athletes reported increasing fatigue that manifested in a certain lack of motivation.

Tips for an iron-rich diet

The body can ingest iron from animal products (fish, meat) two times better than iron from vegetable products. Therefore, endurance athletes should only fprgo meat and fish if they consistently consume vegetable foods that are rich in iron. In addition, you need to consider supporting and inhibitive factors in your iron intake.

Pflanzliche Eisenquellen

- Amaranth is an ancient crop plant. It is considered one of the oldest crop plants of human kind. It is primarily the seeds of the plant that are used and are reminiscent of millet. Even for the Aztecs, Inca, and Maya, the cereal-like grains (amaranthus caudatus, primarily referred to as *Kiwicha*, this name is still used today in the Andes region) were a staple food along with quinoa and corn. Amaranth is one of the few plants that contain qualitative carbohydrates, protein, and minerals. It can be cooked like rice or mixed with other cereal in the form of amaranth pops. Amaranth can be purchased in health food stores.

- Suggestions for iron in salads: 2 tsp sunflower seeds per person in a skillet, roast lightly without fat; sprinkle the toasted seeds over the finished salad.

- Spinach as a source of iron is overrated. Unfortunately the previous spinach recommendations were based on an analysis error. Please forgo eating spinach several times a week because spinach contains oxalic acid, which negatively affects calcium absorption.

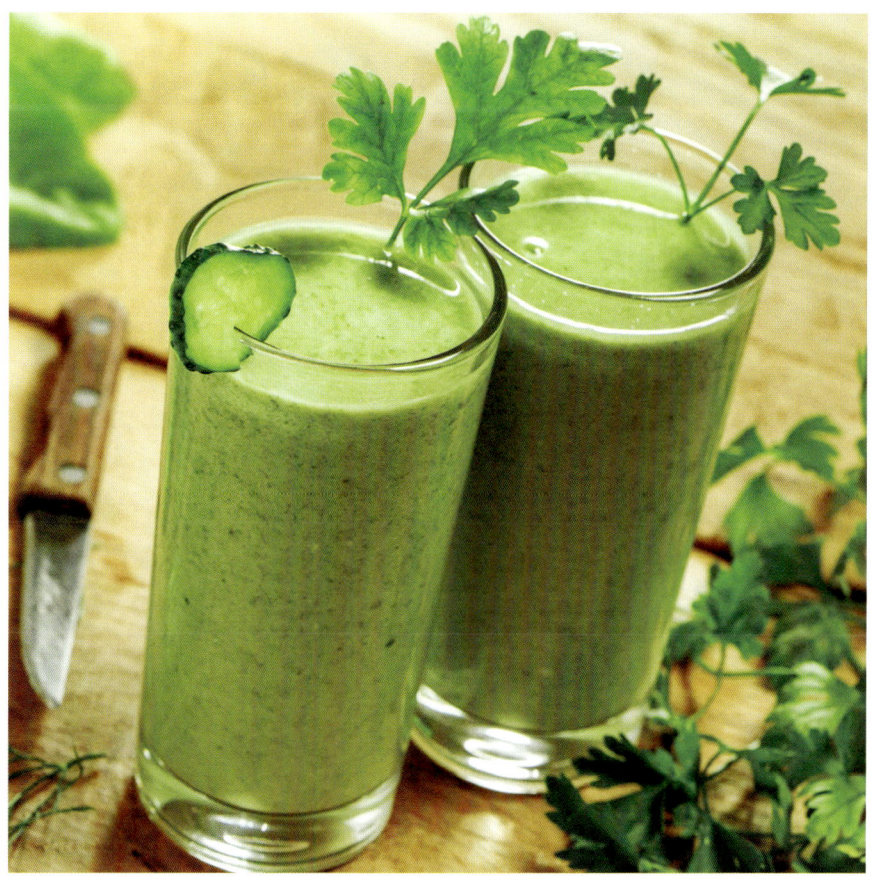

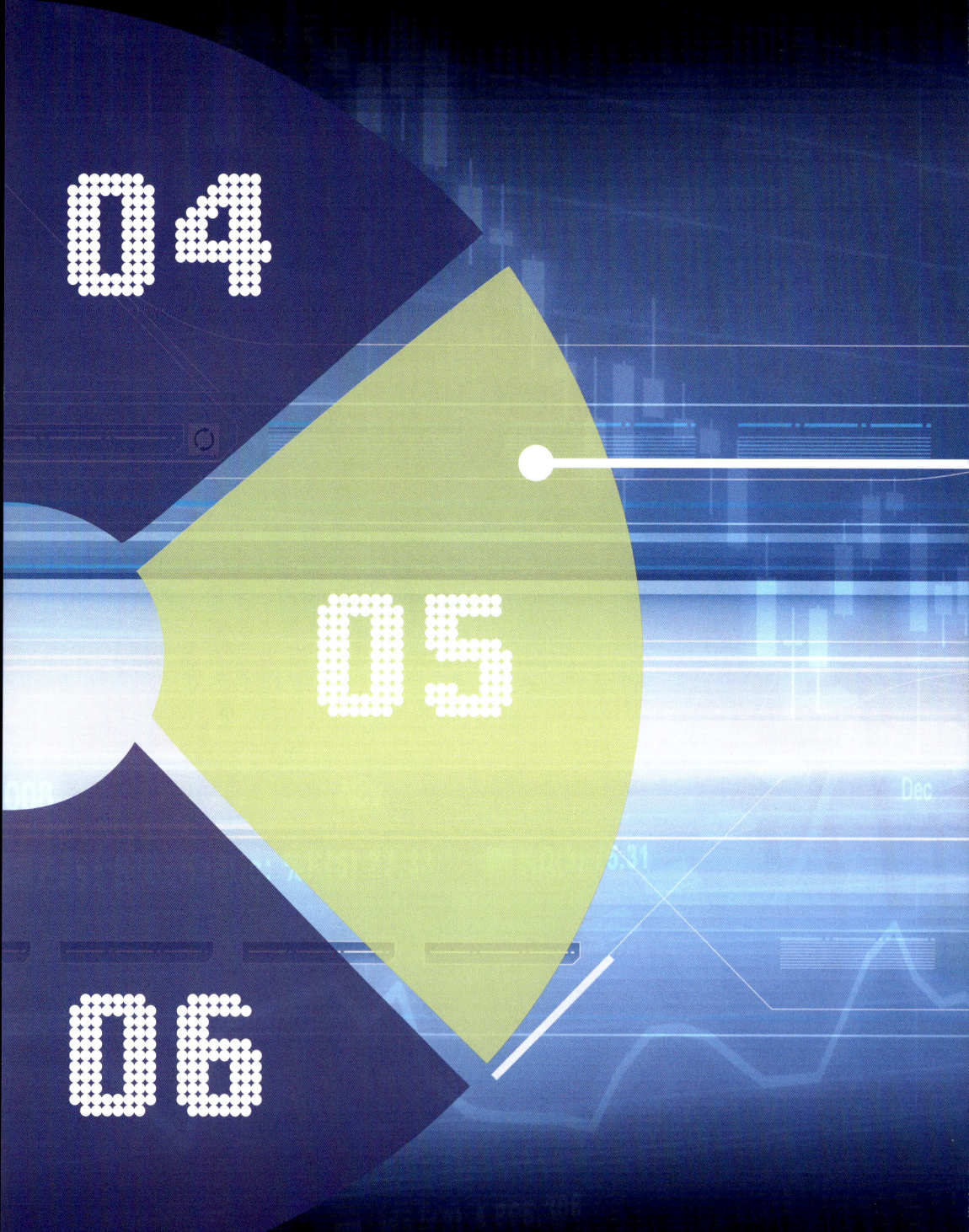

MORE ENERGY
FOR A VITAL LIFE

5 MORE ENERGY FOR A VITAL LIFE

5.1 EXERCISE: FIT INSTEAD OF EXHAUSTED, THE PATH TO MORE ENERGY

MORE ENERGY WITH MODERATE EXERCISE

Overall interest in health-related topics, from executives and highly-engaged professionals, is greater than ever. Ten years ago, many of these people went to fitness studios. But all too often joining a fitness facility appears to have resulted from a heroic decision that turned out to be not very productive. Signing up and then working out regularly are just two separate things. And so it happened that many of the supposedly physically active people in reality were just an index card at the fitness studio or sports club. Top athletic performances to offset professional demands aren't always the best example, either.

For many people it is also apparently difficult to bring more movement into their lives because athletic activity seems to still be very much linked to the achievement principle. Meaning, we put the bar too high and are soon frustrated because we are unable to keep up with the sports enthusiasts who flex their well-formed muscles right next to us in the fitness studio while lifting ever-heavier weights seemingly without effort, or who pass us on the bike trail with their state-of-the-art racing cycles. Many people will ask themselves: Why am I spending my free time struggling and cutting a poor figure, just to go home wiped out and exhausted, with sore muscles to look forward to?

But our experiences in recent years show that executives, in particular, who are under a lot of professional stress, seek a borderline athletic equivalent.

Their motto is "More is more," and nothing is further from the truth. Another maxim is "Use what little time you have intensely."

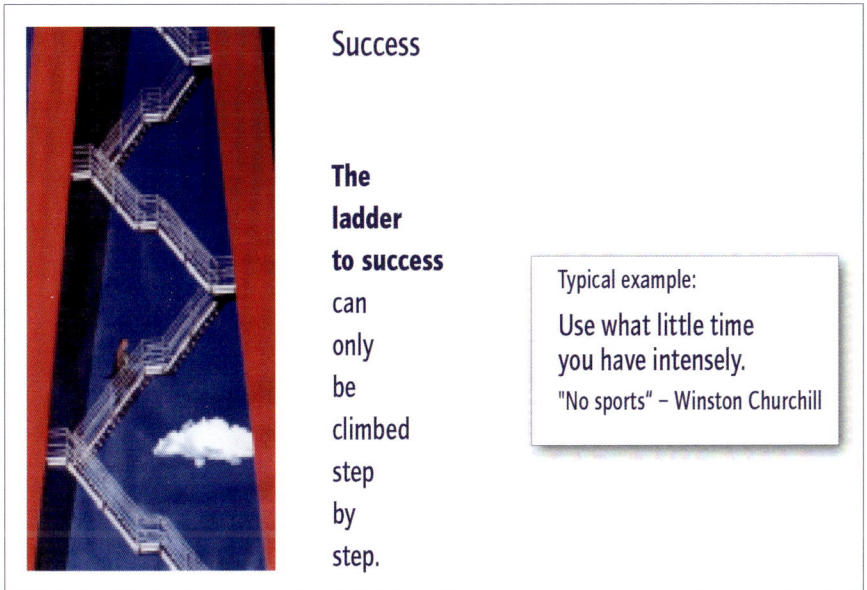

Fig. 52

TOO MUCH IS NOT HEALTHY

The ladder of success must be climbed step by step. Anyone who thinks that he can accomplish top athletic feats in the little time he has to spare is hugely mistaken. Achieving an optimal healthy balance by running three marathons a year is impossible.

In sports, too, the dosage determines whether physical activity promotes health or weakens the body and makes it more vulnerable. The extent to which excessive ambition can be damaging is well documented.

Our experience shows that of the 4,150 executives who worked out intensely three to four times per week and participated in athletic competitions, 75% suffered a heart attack or various types of cancer after 25 years. Their athletic activity as preventative health care was obviously not only ineffective, but even counterproductive.

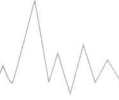 TOP PERFORMANCE IN BUSINESS AND SPORTS

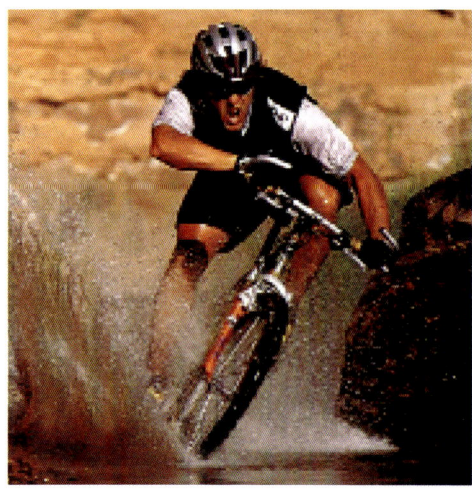

Sports = health – performance capacity?

Photos like this should be a thing of the past.

Anyone who engages in sports recreationally and doesn't want to stress his body further cannot expect it to bring top athletic performances.

Fig. 53

Anyone who wants to perform his athletic activities along the lines of "higher, faster, farther", punishes his body unnecessarily. Even in top athletes the dream of winning the championship, the obsession with success as validation of personal strength, the financially lucrative offers, and the growing mental and physical demands lead to increasing exhaustion, severe performance fluctuations, mood fluctuations, and even to various inexplicable injuries. Here, too, it is important to maintain a balance between workload and rest. "Prescription for Energy" is one of the backbones of mental and physical performance capacity.

BETTER COMMUNICATION IN THE IMMUNE SYSTEM
WITH MODERATE ENDURANCE TRAINING

In short, the positive effects of regular physical activity that is in line with individual physical capacity can be summarized in four points:
- Strengthens the immune system.
- Health risk factors decrease (e.g., high cholesterol, high blood pressure, homocysteine, fibrinogen, lipoprotein a values).

- Increases stress tolerance.
- Increases quality of life in the sense of overall body-mind-spirit well-being.

Our results from 4,150 executives (entrepreneurs, executive managers, executive staff) clearly show that those who engaged in regular moderate endurance training have a considerably lower risk of getting sick. The body's defenses build an extremely complicated system that meets external influences with a variety of reactions. Moderate athletic activity leads to a qualitative improvement of highly proficient immune cells, the *killer cells*. In a well-conditioned person, a high concentration of binding sites can be detected on the surface of these cells that can more effectively attract and destroy viruses and pathogens and also tumor cells. This effect of a heightened sensitization of the immune cells is caused primarily by stimulation via certain messenger substances, the *interleukins*, whose production increases after athletic activity.

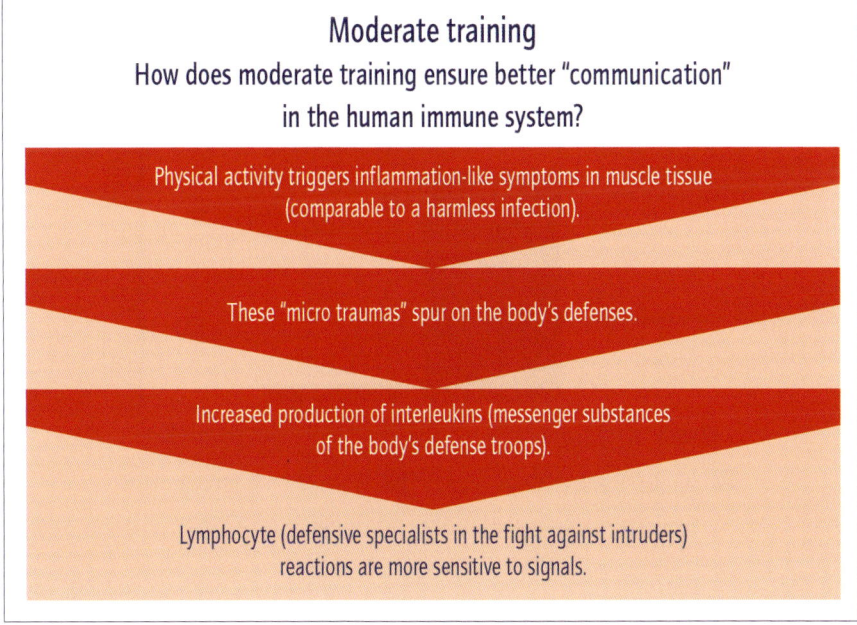

Fig. 54

The internal communication of the immune system is driven by muscular reactions and our body's immune defense shifts to a more active alert state. Fig. 55 shows the chain of signals and reactions triggered inside the organism by moderate exercise that leads to a heightened immune defense.

The more extensive and intense athletic exertion becomes, the higher the risk of getting sick. The infection rate increases with the increasing workload. Of 1,150 top competitive athletes, the 559 athletes who received individually-adapted micronutrient formulas (Prescription for Energy) showed an infection rate of only 4.2% within a two-year time period, while the other 591 athletes showed an infection rate of 54.3% (see fig. 55). The dietary habits in both groups differed only slightly. This result is based on more then 1,000 completed nutrition analyses.

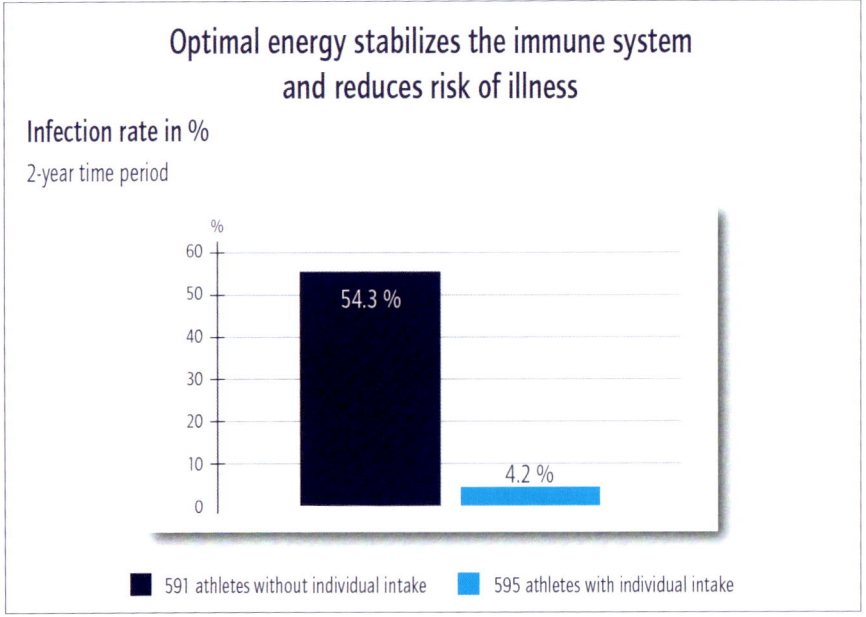

Fig. 55

EXERCISE FOR CALMNESS AND CONFIDENCE: THE BEST STRESS REDUCER

This is certainly true for moderate physical activity, because everyone knows that exhausting sports don't work as long-term stress reducers. Because if you work out often and excessively, certain stress hormones are released, particularly lots of adrenaline. So you might feel subjectively well because your vegetative nervous system is "hyped up", but you are unable to find real inner peace and relaxation. In the long-term this even has a damaging effect on your health. Conditions such as anxiety, pent up aggressions, and tension can be reduced via moderate endurance training of 3 x 40 min. per week. No medicine has a more positive effect on your personal state—and all that guaranteed without harmful side effects (see fig. 56).

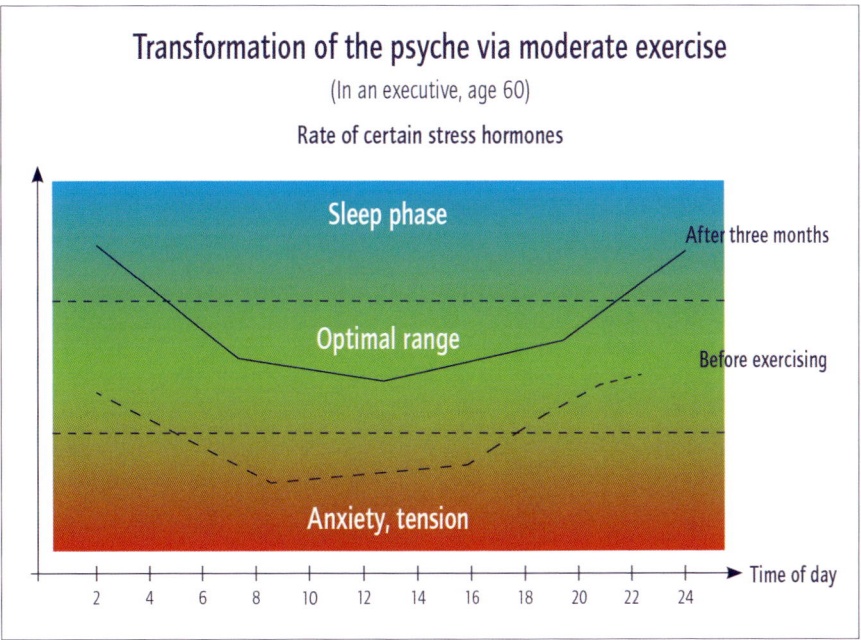

Fig. 56

IN THE GREEN ZONE DURING THE DAY

The color graphic illustration (fig. 56) of the composition of different stress hormones in the course of the day means: Phases in the blue zone are preferable during the night, while values should lie in the green zone during the day. Red phases are not a good prerequisite for creativity and are harmful to your health. Green phases at night indicate strong activity of your vegetative nervous system, which is also not so good because you are unable to regenerate from the daytime stresses. An individual stress profile can be created (see fig. 85, pg. 154) with simple saliva sampling (4-5 samples).

THE BEST EXERCISE FOR YOUR BRAIN (LIFE KINETIK®) – ALWAYS NEW MOVEMENT PATTERNS

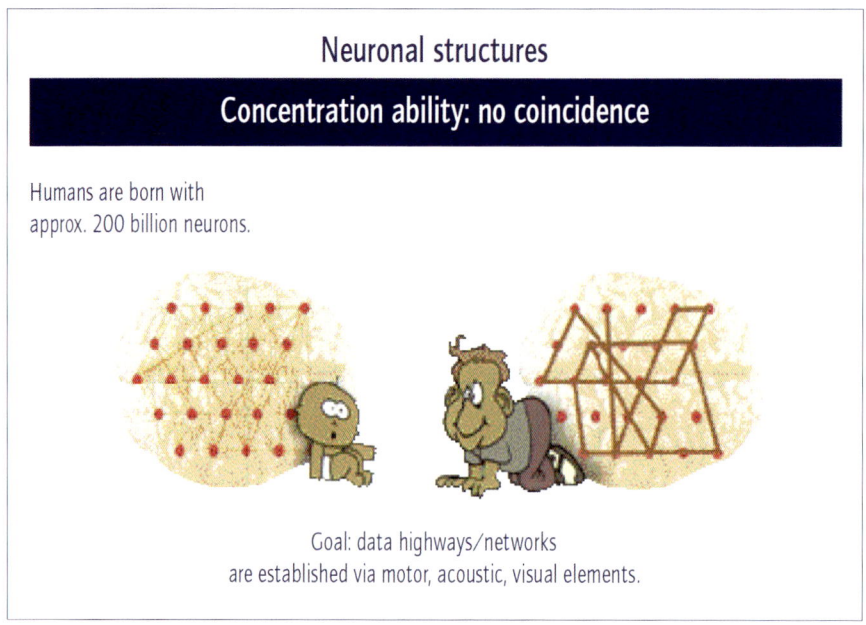

Fig. 57

Life Kinetik® benefits your body in developing the brain's reserves, meaning better performance by tapping into reserves in the structural, biochemical, and intellectual areas to create the best preconditions for daily thought processes and tasks in everyday life and sports. Since this training involves little physical exertion, it provides support to everyone in his personal development, regardless of age and fitness level. Just one hour per week is enough to see initial changes after just a short time. Many former and active elite athletes from alpine skiing, biathlon, soccer, handball, and tennis backgrounds already benefit today from this once-a-week training.

As our stress hormone analyses with ambitious golfers show: The once-a-week 45-minute use brought about such a considerable performance boost in these golfers that they were able to set course records. Regular cortisol measurements (stress hormone) document that significant stress reduction can be achieved with Life Kinetik®, which in turn can clearly improve cognitive performance capacity. You can find out more about the training content of this successful training at www.LifeKinetik.de. There you can also find trainers in your region.

A human being is born with approximately 200 billion neurons. The best method for cross-linking these neuronal structures is the execution of specific movements that can simultaneously activate different areas of the brain (see fig. 58).

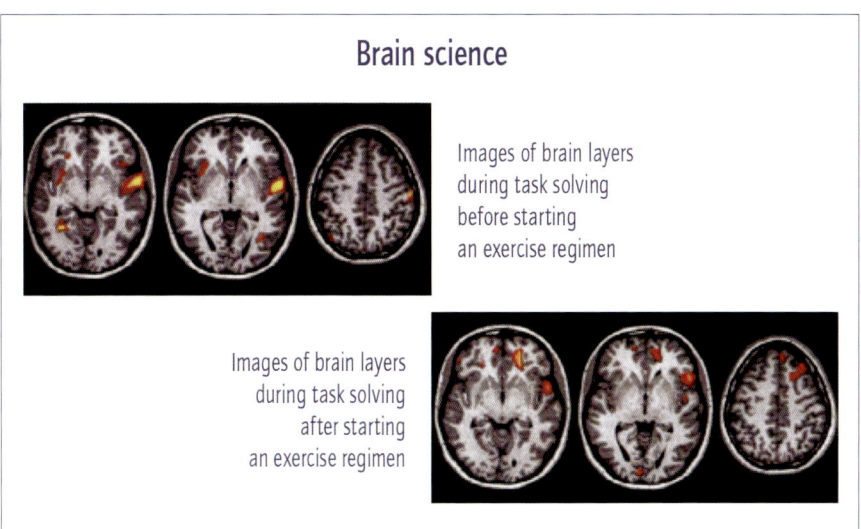

Fig. 58

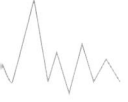

Our practical experience shows that people who regularly engage in this type of movement training considerably improve their intellectual farsightedness via conscious perception, grasp coherences in discussions more quickly, and better and more attentively track visual things in their professional settings.

Top competitive athletes benefit from these various movement tasks. They reduce their energy and strength requirements, achieve an elegant and harmonic execution of difficult motion sequences, and improve their spatial perception and orientation. A daily five-minute coordinative training with elements of Life Kinetik® can result in definite changes to crosslinking in many neuronal structures (see fig. 58).

STRESS MEASURE: YOUR PULSE RATE

Walking without panting was once the motto for healthy movement. But it isn't quite that simple because, depending on the type of sport and temperatures, you can overload yourself and not notice in time. Measuring the pulse rate is therefore imperative in order to engage in well-dosed exercise. Someone who burns approximately 2,000 kcal in the form of athletic activity achieves optimal exercise for health. A 90 kg man doing a 30-minute extensive endurance run burns about 400 kcal.

How to test your load capacity

You can determine your optimal heart rate for exercise with this simple test. Albeit, it isn't as accurate as a professional load capacity analysis performed in a specialized institute, but it is helpful for getting started. You will need a heart rate monitor and a good pair of well-fitting running shoes, as well as a level practice route.

Determining the optimal heart rate

- Create a test log using the following layout:

  Resting heart rate   BPM
  Heart rate w/4-count breathing rhythm   BPM
  Heart rate w/3-count breathing rhythm   BPM

- Measure your resting heart rate: Sit down and relax for 3 minutes, and then take your pulse with the heart rate monitor and write down the result in your test log.

- Walk 4 steps while inhaling once. Take another 4 steps while exhaling once. Practice this four-count breathing rhythm for 5 minutes.

- Now increase your speed as long as you are able to maintain the four-count rhythm. After walking for 10 minutes, measure your heart rate and record it in your test log. The pulse you take in this manner is the target heart rate that you should aim for in future workouts.

- Increase your walking/running speed so that you inhale or exhale every 3 steps you take. With this three-count breathing rhythm you will reach a load intensity that an unfit person initially cannot even maintain for 5 minutes. Record your heart rate at this intensity level after about 5 minutes of walking or running.

- Working out at a two-count breathing rhythm should be avoided: They result in additional activation of the vegetative nervous system and increase the stress level in tense people.

HOW TO TRAIN CORRECTLY

Once you have done a load analysis, you are ready to start your personal workout program.

This is how it works
Choose the four-count breathing rhythm while you are walking and aim for the target heart rate your ascertained in your load analysis. If you get winded, you are going too fast. The motto is: Succeed without panting! In this manner you avoid exhaustion and greatly improve your performance capacity, stress tolerance, and quality of life within only eight weeks.

While previously sedentary people initially walk, physically active people will probably already run in order to reach their target rate. The speed and the distance covered are completely irrelevant. What matters is the amount of exercise time. Start by exercising 3 x per week for 30-40 minutes each (e.g., Monday, Wednesday, Friday); later you can run every day if you like.

The level of your personal optimal heart rate also depends on the type of sport. Therefore you cannot simply transfer the target heart rate you just ascertained to another form of exercise. For cycling and skiing, the heart rates are about 8-10% lower and for swimming, because of the effects of the mammalian diving reflex, 6-7% lower than for running.

After just a few weeks of exercising you will no longer reach your target heart rate at the same speed. Now you have to increase your speed to be able to "home in" on your old pulse rate. It is best if you track your progress with the help of an exercise journal. In this journal you can record your resting heart rate that should be measured prior to each workout and that can be subject to fluctuations (e.g., due to a slight illness, insufficient fluid intake, cigarette smoking, overheating due to warm seasonal temperatures or warm clothing, spending time in higher elevations in the mountains).

FOR THOSE WHO LOVE THAT ATHLETIC KICK, PROFESSIONAL LOAD ANALYSIS MAKES SENSE

If you absolutely need that kick of athletic limit workloads, we recommend paying attention to the following aspects during a professional check-up:

- Exercise electrocardiogram, if possible with echocardiography
- Measure thyroid hormone level (Caution: No intense workout the day before because this may cause a stress-induced rise in thyroid hormone levels)
- Complete blood panel, also with secondary risk factors Lp(a) and homocysteine, CrP level, HbA1c long-term glucose level, liver, and kidney levels, ferritin, intracellular micronutrient analysis Mg, Zn, ferritin, vitamin B_9 and B_{12}
- Testing of the functional energy metabolism as indicator of impaired activity of certain enzymes
- Stress ergometric exam on a treadmill or bike with metabolism analysis (lactate) or alternative spiroergometry
- Biochemical function analysis (measuring strength in legs, abdominals, back);
- Personal training with practical suggestions
- Individualized formula based on the special blood and urine analysis

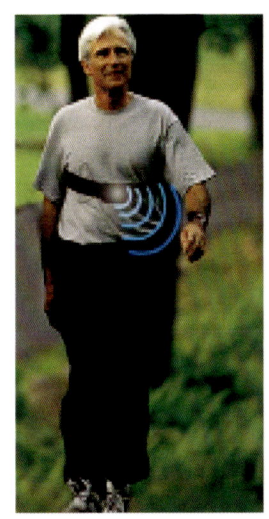
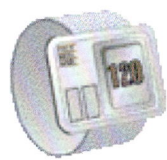

Measuring the heart rate

Heart rate monitor with wireless transmission of frequency

The heart rate is measured via a wireless transmission principle by transferring the heart rate from the ribcage area to a heart rate monitor at the wrist.

Fig. 59

5.2 BRAIN FOOD FOR EXECUTIVES

A human brain makes up only 2% of total body weight, but requires 20% of the overall metabolism. The many stressors of our professional lives require a continuous energy supply. The brain is supplied primarily by the circulating blood sugar and possesses almost no glucose storage reserves. High-quality nutritional proteins elevate the mood and boost thinking processes.

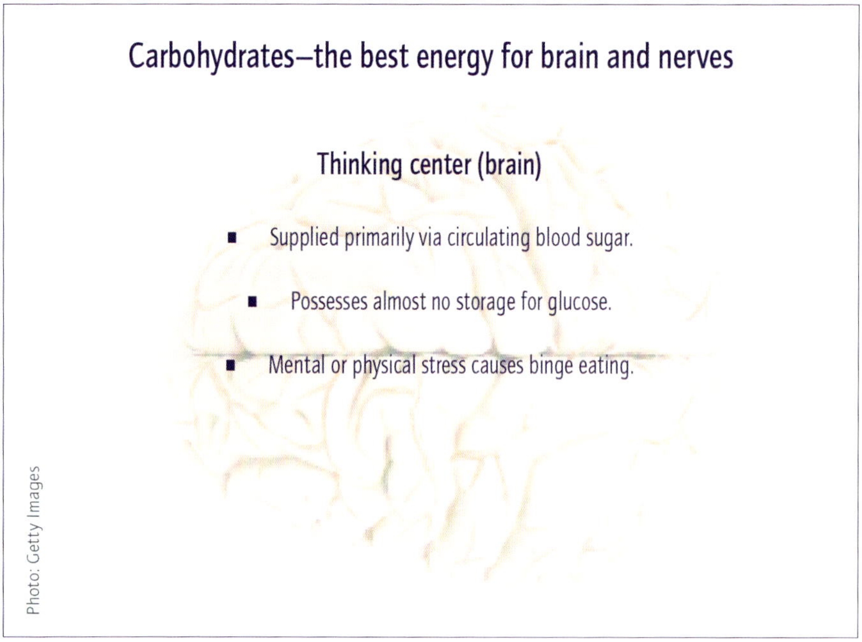

Carbohydrates—the best energy for brain and nerves

Thinking center (brain)

- Supplied primarily via circulating blood sugar.
- Possesses almost no storage for glucose.
- Mental or physical stress causes binge eating.

Photo: Getty Images

Fig. 60

Mental and physical stress causes binge eating and often leads to the uncontrolled consumption of sweets. Here in particular, unsulfured apricots (dried fruit) or fresh pineapple chunks are recommended as direct energy suppliers.

Try not to consume any monosaccharides (simple sugar) to maintain your ability to concentrate during the day. Try not to consume carbohydrates at night.

MORE ENERGY FOR A vital LIFE

Fitness food for the brain

- The brain makes up only 2% of total body weight.
- But it requires 20% of the entire basal metabolism.
- The brain has a daily supply of 1,200 l of blood and 115 g of sugar.
- High-quality nutritional proteins lift the mood and boost thinking processes.

Photo: Getty Images

Fig. 61

These cause a long-term insulin release that can already trigger another binge-eating attack after just half an hour. Please bear in mind: A fresh pineapple has as many calories as 15 gummy bears (see fig. 62).

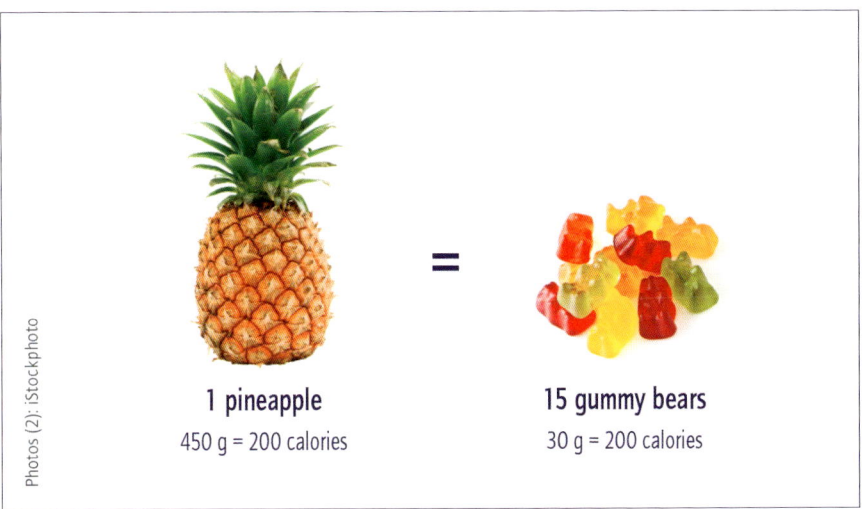

1 pineapple
450 g = 200 calories

15 gummy bears
30 g = 200 calories

Fig. 62

125

Please also be careful not to eat too many white flour products (white pasta, white bread, white rice) because these cause increased acidosis (see fig. 64) and can still cause binge-eating attacks.

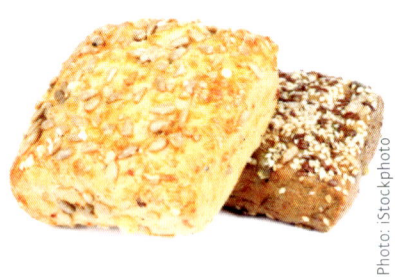

Fig. 63

Who among you is truly able to eat according to the five-meal model during the workday? Of the 4,150 executives hardly anyone was able to adhere to this principle (see fig. 64).

MORE ENERGY FOR A vital LIFE

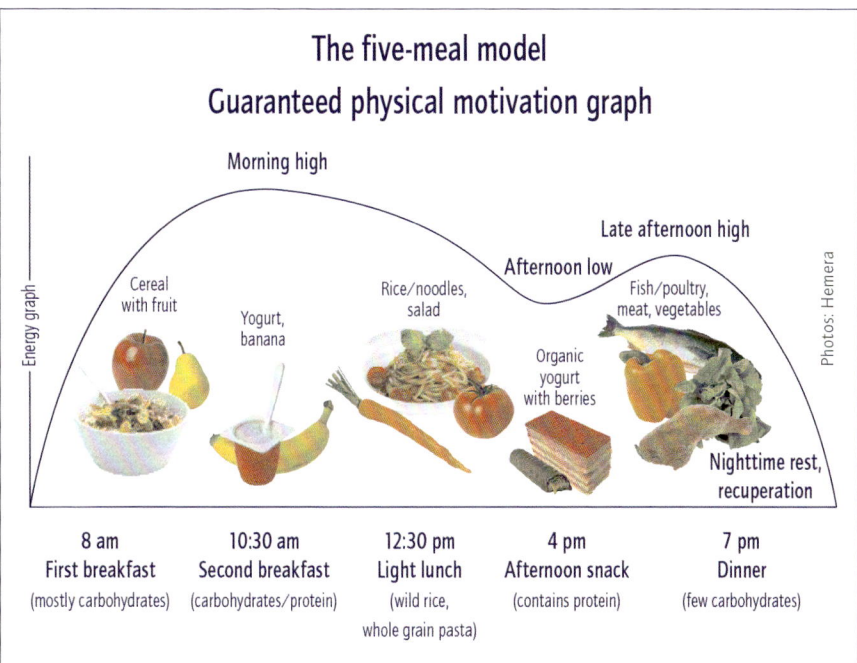

Fig. 64

Often the hectic workday doesn't permit a regular, health-conscious diet. But it is important to know that consuming a lot of protein in the evening does not make for restful sleep because it increasingly activates the vegetative nervous system. The following tips are easy to implement.

Daily nutrition

Morning

Goal: starting energy, overall activation
Breakfast of mostly carbohydrates balanced
with activating protein (phenylalanine, tyrosine)

Second breakfast

Goal: endurance
Carbohydrate and protein snack

Afternoon

Goal: prevent midday low and sleepiness
(Stabilize motivation for the second half of the day)
Light, mostly high-quality protein foods
with high nutrient density, fat only with good judgment)

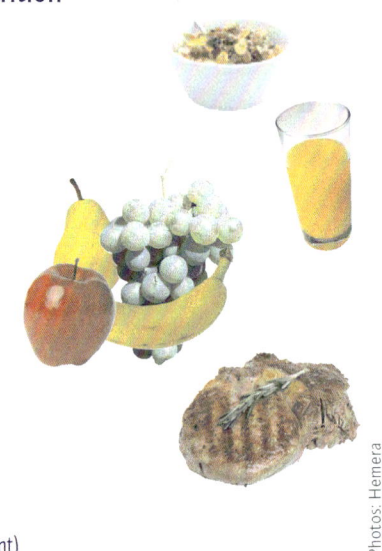

Photos: Hemera

Fig. 65

Therefore optimal meals are...

- Pasta with vegetables
- Rice and vegetable skillet
- Oat flakes with banana

Possible food combinations in the course of a day:

- Breakfast of mostly carbohydrates (e.g., rolled oats with fruit)
- At lunch a small serving of wild rice with vegetables (focus on whole grain products)
- Afternoon snack of organic yogurt with fruit (e.g., blueberries)
- Evening meal of, poultry with vegetables (no carbohydrates)

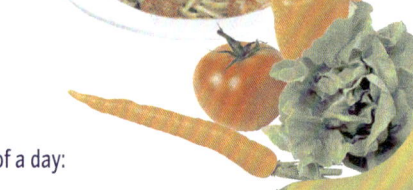

Photos: Hemera

Fig. 66

CHECK YOUR ACID-ALKALINE BALANCE

An optimal acid-alkaline balance is an important prerequisite for the absorption of micronutrients. This acid-alkaline balance can be easily ascertained through a test. You can ascertain your own profile by using pH test strips. You can purchase these test strips with a color-coded chart at any pharmacy.

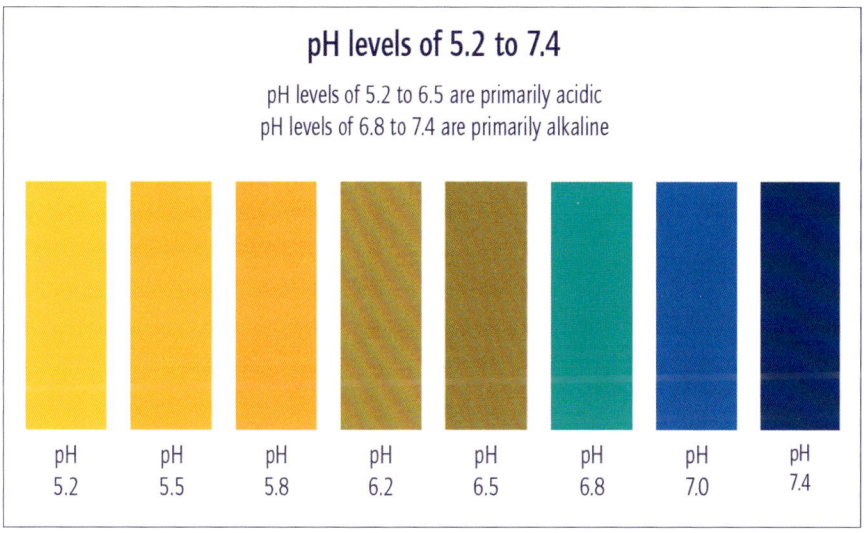

Fig. 67

For measuring in our institute, the executives and athletes receive a three-day journal form. Measuring pH levels should be done in the morning on an empty stomach, in the afternoon, and in the evening before dinner. The correct execution: Hold the test strip midstream under urine and hold for 1 sec. Then use the color scale to determine the result and record it in the journal. In addition also record your state of well-being on the test form. You can find a download code for the journal form in PDF format on pg. 218. You can use this to record your individual results (see fig. 68). We recommend doing this test only on weekdays, as it is our experience that diets change somewhat on weekends.

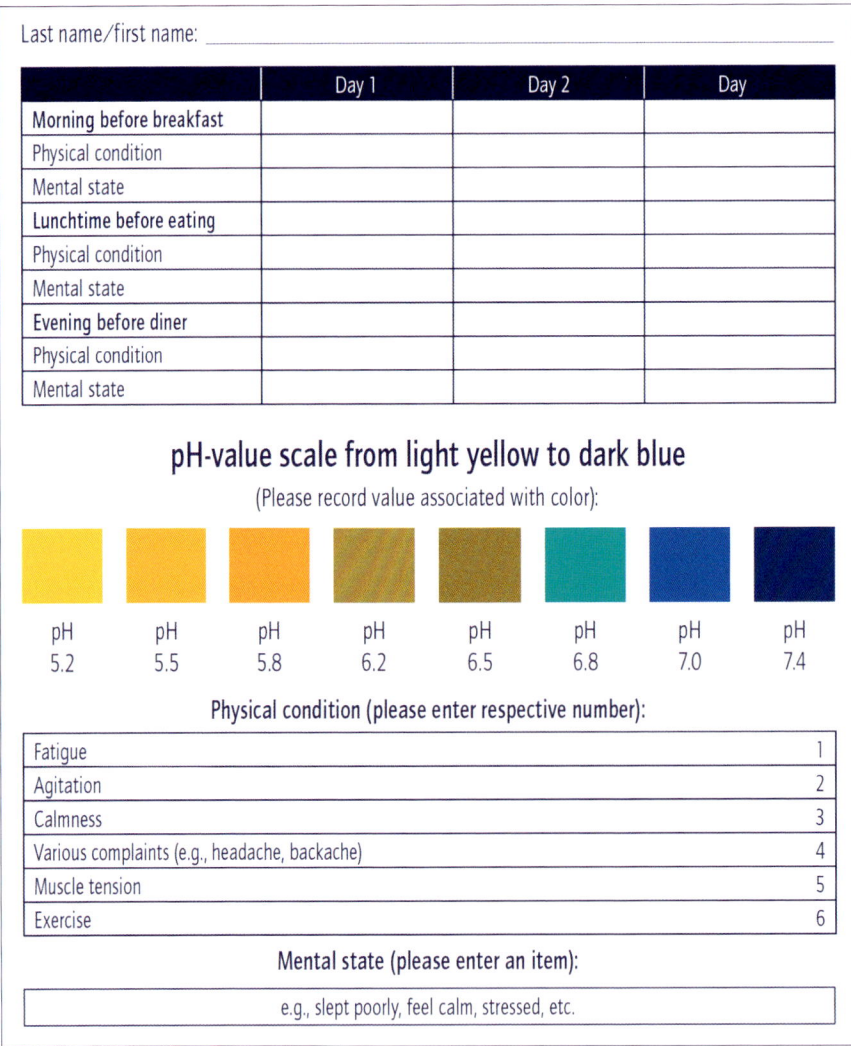

Fig. 68

If the pH values from the three-day acid-alkaline profiles are < 6.5, the targeted intake of an alkaline powder would be sensible. In any case, reduce the intake of sweets and white flour products since these can result in diet-related acidosis. Complete regular journal measurements. Increasing acidosis verifiably also raises the risk of injury to the stressed connective tissue structures in athletes.

TIPS AND ADVICE FOR ATHLETES

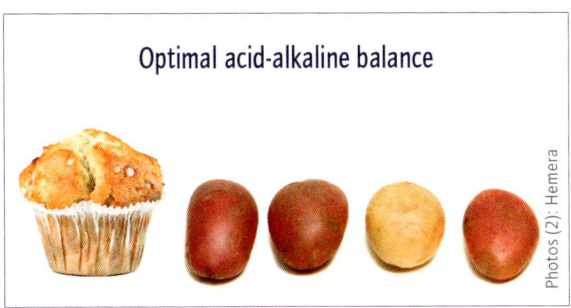

Fig. 69

Acid and base foods in our nutrition

1:4 is the approximate ratio of acids to bases as it also occurs naturally in the body. To achieve this ratio we really only need to know what produces acidity and what produces alkalinity. Many acid producers can easily be replaced by healthier foods. For instance, instead of polished rice you can use much more tasty, unpeeled rice.

Important advice

For competitive athletes: White pasta and white rice are favorite meals. On training days, try to eat primarily whole grain pasta or wild rice, as these do not cause additional acidosis. However, please do not eat whole grain pasta (rice) on competition days, as the retention time in the gastrointestinal tract is too long.

Please ensure a regular intake of non-insulin dependent sugar such as galactose and ribose (1 tsp each before and after athletic exertion, also see chapter 6.2).

We basically differentiate four food groups with respect to their impact on our acid-alkaline balance.

Alkaline foods

These include primarily

- Potatoes
- Vegetables
- Herbs like parsley, chives, marjoram, thyme, paprika, dill, oregano
- Fruit
- Raw milk
- Uncarbonated mineral water

Neutral foods

They maintain the balance between acids and bases. They include:

- Butter
- Walnuts
- Straight vegetable oils
- Tap water

Acidic foods

These are foods that do not contain acids but who produce them during processing in the metabolism:

- Sugar,
- Sugary sweets (marzipan, chocolate, cake, ice cream)
- All peeled or polished grains and their products, also mixed wheat and rye bread
- Lemonade containing sugar, white flour products (breads, pasta, polished rice)
- Coffee
- Alcoholic beverages

Acidity suppliers

These are protein-containing foods that also have an excess of acidic minerals (sulphur, phosphorus, iodine, chlorine). In some cases their consumption produces additional acids during metabolization. In this way excessive meat consumption doubles the loss of alkalinity. These include:

- Meat and innards (liver, heart, kidneys, brain),
- Poultry (chicken, duck, goose, turkey),
- Game (rabbit, venison, wild boar),
- Eggs (only yokes are alkaline),
- Cheese, Greek yogurt,
- Meat broth.

FLUID BALANCE: OPTIMAL–SMART–EFFECTIVE

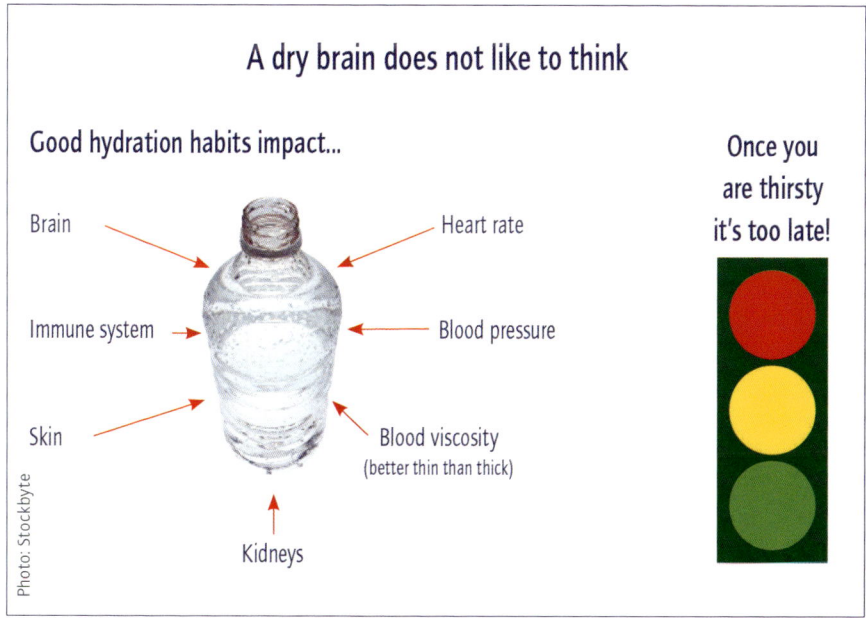

Fig. 70

Effective hydration with alkaline beverages

Mineral water: sodium content > 350 mg, but less than 1,000 mg

The greater the mineral water's bicarbonate concentration
(hydrogen carbonate), the better excess acid
can be transferred to the blood.

Bicarbonate concentration: at least > 500 mg
Optimal > 1,500 mg in uncarbonated water without carbonic acid

Sodium-rich hydration in sports

- Quick carbohydrate absorption
- Quick water absorption
- Little urine excretion

Fig. 71

Faster recovery with smart drinking and eating after athletic exertion

Faster regeneration takes place with targeted replenishing of stressed glycogen stores
in liver and muscles within the first two hours after exertion.

Phase 1: Immediately after competition or training.

Regeneration beverage: recovery drink

- Combination of galactose/ribose (1 tsp before and after training)
- Please no more than 500 ml at one time, otherwise absorption decreases
- Carbohydrate share 35-70 g per l (approx. 3-7%)
  all beverages above 8% block gastric emptying speed (e.g., Coca-Cola with 11%)
- Sodium content above 350 mg/l
  (1 fizzy potassium citrate tablet from a pharmacy 750 mg)
- Supplement or mix with a good uncarbonated mineral water
- Protein content approx. 20-25 g per l

Fig. 72

MORE ENERGY FOR A vital LIFE

Important tips about hydration

- Once you are thirsty it's way too late.

- Increase fluid intake slowly so gastrointestinal receptors can adapt to more liquid.

- The gastrointestinal tract cannot absorb more than > 500 ml of fluid.

- Please bear in mind the quality of mineral water as previously described.

- Taking magnesium during athletic exertion is not advisable because it places too much stress in the gastrointestinal tract, and this may result in intolerance.

Fig. 73

Diet for a training day

Get-fit breakfast (high in carbohydrates)

- 5 tbs of rolled oats or whole grain cereal
- 3 tbs of wheat germ, 1 banana sliced, with yogurt and with vanilla flavor (if desired), with that a glass of freshly-squeezed orange juice
- Before training 1 tsp galactose/ribose

1. Training

During training drink approx. 500 ml (sports drink mixed with high-quality mineral water, as previously described) (Optimal sodium-hydrogen carbonate share).

Immediately after training:

- After training 1 tsp galactose/ribose, 2-3 heaping tbs AM-Formula blend, stirred into 200 ml juice and drink (fills the amino acid pools and stabilizes connective tissue).

Fig. 74

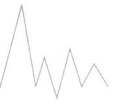

Lunch
From the accompanying carb-loading chart (beneficial food combinations)

Optimal and quick recovery with carbohydrates, potassium, chromium, and high-quality protein combination.

Example:

- 3-4 potatoes
- 125 g Greek yogurt, seasonal herbs, salt, and pepper
- Seasonal salad with fresh champignon mushrooms
- 1-2 eggs
- Dessert: ½ fresh pineapple or a small fruit salad (kiwi, banana, etc.)

Afternoon snack
For in between: high-quality cereal bars, fruit tart, etc.

Fig. 75

Dinner
Carb loading from the skillet (pasta or rice-vegetable dish)
Simple homemade meal

Optimal and quick recovery with carbohydrates, potassium, chromium, and high-quality protein combination.
Whole grain pasta or wild rice contains silicic acid, which stabilizers of tendons and ligaments.

- 150 g of wild rice or whole grain pasta, cook for 15 min.

- Next put approx. 150 g of frozen vegetables in a skillet with 1 tbs of oil, add rice or pasta, and stir in skillet with vegetables for about 6-8 min.

Fig. 76

> ## A few tips
>
> - 1-2 hours before exertion: for instance white bread with lots of honey or jam, no butter.
>
> - Also mild, ripe, base-friendly fruit:
>   melons, mangos, or pears;
>   no unripe fruit, because it takes too long to digest.
>
> - No competition or training without breakfast—better get up earlier.
>
> - Practice more efficient hydration—only then can you implement this during competitions.
>
> - Daily intake of oranges, kiwi, and grapefruit, keep your connective tissue young.
>
> - Avoid eating a lot of sweets and white flour products (white noodles, white rice), and lots of meat and cold cuts, because these cause overacidification in the metabolism and block absorption of important minerals.
>
> - The first two hours after exertion determine your regeneration time
>   (optimal behavior, particularly
>   with respect to diet, ensures success).

Fig. 77

OPTIMAL CARBOHYDRATE STRATEGY: SUPER CARB LOADING

Effective modern super carb loading involves food combinations that are high in carbohydrates, potassium, and chromium, while also supplying protein. These food combinations are recommended especially during the final days leading up to a competition and immediately after training and competitions.

The bulk of energy derived from the super carb loading meals should always come from carbohydrates. When assembling the meals, the carbohydrate portion should always be dominant. In addition, complex carbohydrates should often be of the whole grain variety. Only on competition days are white noodles and rice recommended because due to their respective dietary fiber, whole grain products remain in the digestive tract longer (see fig. 78).

Please note:
Use the accompanying chart to create
your personal food combination.

Super carb loading

- Carbohydrates must be dominant!

- Carbohydrates should be whole grain:
  whole grain pasta, whole grain rice, whole grain bread.

- Do not eat whole grain pasta, on competition days (do eat white pasta, because these are easier to digest).

- Organic foods: use potato peels which are optimal for building connective tissue.

Fig. 78

Nothing works without carbohydrates!
Food combinations that contain carbohydrates, potassium, chromium, while also supplying protein.

Super carb loading

Carbohydrate-rich foods	Potassium-rich foods	Chromium-rich foods	Protein-rich foods
Pasta	Tomato soup	Mushrooms	Low-fat cheese
Rice	Vegetables	Mushroom gravy	Peas, turkey
Bread	Tomatoes, peppers	Edam cheese	
Potatoes	Greek yogurt		Greek yogurt, eggs
Cereal	Fruit	Rolled oats, nuts	Low-fat milk, yogurt

Fig. 79: From Feil/Wessinghage Nutrition and Training

5.3 ENJOYING LIFE WITHOUT BEING STRESSED

EVERYTHING GETS EASIER WHEN YOU ARE RELAXED

Strength lies in calmness. Sure, but how to find that calmness when there is chaos? The psyche also needs to be taken care of so everyday stresses don't overwhelm us.

Active strategies for stress relief
Everyone complains about being stressed, meaning that they have too much on his plate. In professional life, it is practically an expectation to be stressed as the mark of an engaged, dynamic executive.

Our results from 4,150 executives show that 70% are unable to wind down after work and feel extremely stressed (see fig. 7, pg. 18). Every individual can clearly improve his performance capacity and the associated creativity with the concept for success: Prescription for Energy. We already described the status quo of the overall energy metabolism and the positive changes with individualized micronutrient formulas on pages 22 and 23. Of course this also applies to top competitive athletes who are constantly pushing the limits of mental and physical stress.

Body and soul suffer
But we cannot continue to intake more "energy" for the long-term, even if it is truly lacking, and at the same time manage our existing resources irresponsibly. For this reason strategies for stress relief are a very useful addition. You can learn to be calm and relaxed. The dramatic trend in recent years towards increasing chronic fatigue syndrome in executives, top competitive athletes shows the urgent need for action. But you should most definitely also utilize the many available relaxation methods and learn which one is the right fit for you so you can then tackle the challenges with renewed emotional vigor.

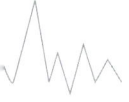

TOP PERFORMANCE IN BUSINESS AND SPORTS

Rarely can we spontaneously transport ourselves from a stressful situation to an idyllic rural setting or simply home to our beds. Relaxation techniques are a way to find a peaceful place within ourselves during times of great tension.

Fig. 80: Agitation, and aggression—good mood, and creative—sleepy, and mentally run down

THE DIFFERENT METHODS

There are many relaxation methods for you to choose from. Some techniques have proven particularly successful because they are easy to learn and can be implemented without much preparation when they are most needed—namely in a stressful situation or for a quick refresher in between.

In addition, to make a choice, it is important to know what type you are. Some people can relax best through the power of their thoughts, while some require conscious sensory perception, yet others need targeted physical exercises. Find out what is the easiest way for you to achieve inner harmony! But all of the techniques have one thing in common: You must practice them for a time to be able to apply them successfully.

Autogenic training

Autogenic training is not a good fit for impatient people, because it takes several weeks before you are able to effectively use the exercises. But it can have a deep and long-lasting effect beyond the actual practice time and impact many mental vegetative disorders, such as insomnia. For many people this classic relaxation technique is an effective method against exhaustion, anxiety, or problems concentrating or sleeping. By focusing the mind on certain body regions, muscle tension, breathing, circulation, and cardiac activity can be influenced autosuggestively. Major advantage: It can be practiced anywhere in any situation, if you know how.

Actually you need nothing more than to assume a relaxed seated or reclined position and mentally repeat some proven suggestive formulas ("my right arm is very heavy, warm, etc.") in a certain rhythm. Theoretically this technique can be learned from an instructional book. But in reality it usually requires a lot more practice before the autosuggestion really works. When first getting started, an experienced instructor is also very helpful to guide you through the intrinsically simple exercises, should you choose this method.

Progressive muscle relaxation

This clever relaxation concept was developed by the physiologist Edmund Jacobson at Harvard University. In a seated or reclined position, tense individual muscle groups one by one from toes to forehead for 5-10 sec. and then relax them for 20-30 sec. This method increases sensitivity for muscle tension and develops the ability to consciously relax the muscles.

After practicing this for an extended period of time you achieve a deep mental and physical state of relaxation. The "trick" is: every tensing up is followed by a relaxation phase with less tonicity, breathing is deeper and slower, blood vessels dilate, and heart rate and blood pressure drop.

Progressive muscle relaxation is easy to learn and can be practiced alone. But in the beginning it is helpful to have another person give instructions as to which muscles to target in which order, and how long to maintain the state of muscle tension or relaxation. There are excellent CD's available commercially with which you can practice until you have memorized your program and have developed a sense of timing for the duration of each individual exercise.

Meditation

To many, meditation sounds a bit pretentious and reminiscent of Far Eastern guru wisdom. But mediation means nothing other than inner spiritual contemplation that can take place in many different forms. Not only is it a proven relaxation method, but it can also promote creativity, concentration ability, memory and mental agility, and, for instance, help with insomnia, anxiety, headaches, or increasing depressive moods.

The purpose of meditation is to move the flood of thoughts in your head into a quiet place, to block out the problems and challenges of the day, and to gradually transcend the everyday level of consciousness. The goal is a completely relaxed, but mentally wide-awake, state. Don't become impatient if it doesn't work right away. For many of us, internal contemplation is at first a very unfamiliar state.

Focusing on the breath

This can be the first step to meditation or the form of meditation itself. Conscious "listening" to one's own breathing is an excellent way to achieve mental peace. Close your eyes and focus on the rhythm and feel of your breath without forcing it. Just breathe slowly and evenly, and as you do so notice how the breath flows within you. Focus completely on this process and don't become irritated by your wandering thoughts. It is quite possible that you remember just now something important you have to take care of. Don't fight these distractions, but also don't follow this train of thought any further.

The breath is closely linked to our mental state: when we are upset or scared we automatically breathe faster, or we hold our breath. Conscious slow breathing helps us regain inner peace and emotional evenness.

Visualization and imagery

These forms of meditation can be practiced regardless of place and time. First try to separate yourself internally from the problems at hand and any pressing thoughts and begin to relax by breathing calmly. Tap into your imagination and imagine a pleasant scenario. This can be the memory of a happy experience or even a daydream. Here for once you can indulge in unbridled wishful thinking.

The only thing that is important is that you put yourself completely into that situation, imagine and enjoy every detail. Use all of your senses to do so. During a dream stroll through a flowering meadow in summer, pay close attention to the various colors and shapes of the flowers, take note of the buzzing insects and singing birds, and enjoy the smell of the grass and the wonderful feeling of a soft summer breeze caressing your skin.

You can limit your wishful thinking to a snapshot, or expand it to an entire journey. What's important is that the intensity of your imagination takes you completely away from the here and now to a satisfied, relaxed state of complete physical and emotional well-being. If necessary, consult the experts.

Shaking off tension

A few breathing exercises here and there refresh you like a short slumber and, if necessary, can be done in the restroom during a break from a meeting. Of course it would be better if you could go outside to do this in the fresh air. The following breathing exercise helps to release inner tension and to become physically calm in severely stressful situations.

- Stand tall in a slight straddle and inhale deeply through the nose; count to 5 as you do this.
- Exhale forcefully though the mouth. As you do this, let your arms, shoulders, and upper body fall forward and bend your knees slightly.
- When you inhale again, count to 10. As you do this, straighten your legs and slowly roll your upper body back up, vertebrae by vertebrae, into an upright position. Finally raise your chin.
- Once you are back in an upright position, exhale briefly and start from the beginning. Repeat 3-4 times.

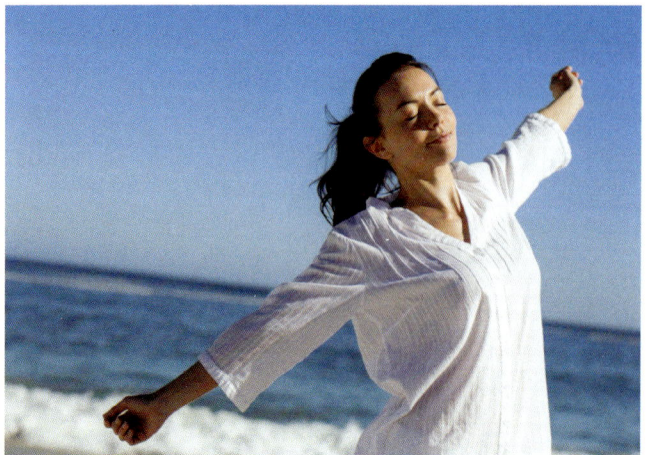

Fig. 81

5.4 HEALTHY AND SOUND SLEEP

SLEEPING LIKE A LOG

You can only dream of that? You and many others—more than 3 million Germans—permanently suffer from insomnia. It affects the ability to concentrate and perform, not to mention causes a bad mood after a restless night. Intensive nocturnal rest is an elixir for physical and mental health, fitness, and memory. Our research shows: 70% of 10,270 entrepreneurs, executives, and executive staff, and 52% of all top competitive athletes have major problems with sleep. The targeted intake of magnesium and L-tryptophan (see pg. 82-83) at a dosage based on blood test results has resulted in a greatly improved sleep quality. You will now learn the importance of sleep for you and the effect it has on, for instance, the immune system.

THE GUARDIAN OF THE IMMUNE SYSTEM

Scientists agree that sufficient sleep strengthens the immune system and promotes better regeneration. A lot happens particularly during the dreamless deep sleep phases. Many hormones are produced to replenish depleted stores; the growth hormone serotonin helps to repair defective cells, and the immune system creates new defensive molecules against pathogens. The brain and nerves recover from the many stimuli and impulses that flood them throughout the day. New studies show that insufficient sleep impairs immunological memory (i.e., the immune system's ability to recognize and neutralize a pathogen). Researchers in Lübeck, Germany injected test subjects with weakened hepatitis A pathogens to provoke an immune response. Vaccinated subjects who were kept awake during the night produced significantly fewer antibodies against the virus in the blood than the sleeping control group. This coincides with the observation that people who are sick appear to instinctively sleep longer and deeper to strengthen their immune defense.

HOW MUCH SLEEP DOES A HUMAN REQUIRE?

The average German goes to bed at 11 pm and sleeps approximately 7 hours. That doesn't mean much because the optimal amount of sleep is an individual quantity that differs from person to person. Babies sleep 16-18 hours per day. From infancy to adolescence the amount of sleep gradually decreases to approximately eight to nine hours, while very old people often only sleep four hours during the night, but then take naps during the day. People who perform hard physical work or extremely stressed adults need more sleep than rested vacationers. So it is less important how many hours you have slept than how rested and refreshed you feel afterward. Over time the deep sleep phases get shorter and shallower due to decreasing melatonin production. Age-related sleep problems are trouble falling asleep, waking up frequently throughout the night, waking up early, and shallower and less restorative sleep.

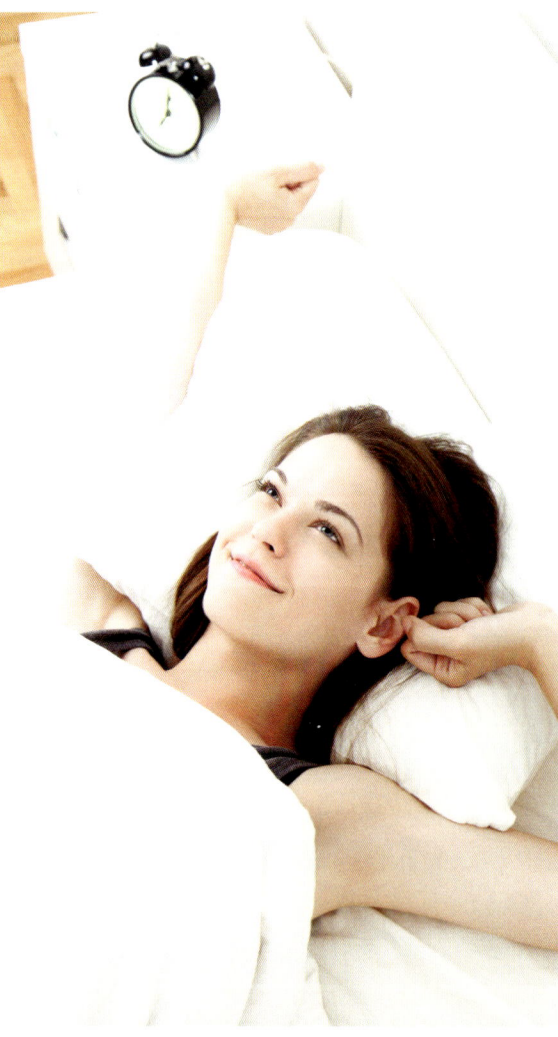

NEW SLEEP SYSTEMS IMPROVE PERFORMANCE CAPACITY

The essence of healthful sleep is of course the bed. Here you should not save in the wrong place. For competitive athletes, and also executives who travel a lot, a good night's sleep is the best regeneration. Better sleep quality reduces the release of stress hormones (cortisol). Our tests results have confirmed this (for additional information on cortisol measurement, see pg. 149).

GROWTH HORMONE: THE MOST IMPORTANT HORMONE OF THE NIGHT

During the night our body switches to another work mode with the objectives for rest and recuperation, and no longer performance. An entire hormone orchestra works during the night to make us fit for the next day. The human growth hormone (HGH) is the most important hormone of the night. It induces formation of new cells that we need every day, provides energy-supplying substances such as fatty acids from the fatty tissue, and degrades the body's waste.

This hormone is particularly important for an athlete's ability to recuperate. When we go to sleep, the pituitary gland starts to produce growth hormone. This production ends in the second half of the night when we no longer have a marked deep sleep phase. This anabolic reaction (rebuilding of stressed protein structures) after intense training or competition-related exertion is a significant guarantor for long-term optimal performance development. Next to an optimal micronutrient supply, sleep quality is the critical factor for regeneration.

The significance of cortisol as a regulating stress hormone

During the first half of the night cortisol is barely detectable. Around 3 am, the cortisol level rises considerably and does so regardless of whether we sleep or not. This hormone is directly controlled by the internal clock. Even if we don't go to sleep until 2 am, the body begins to produce cortisol around 3 am. With the start of increased cortisol production the release of growth hormone from the first half of the night is suppressed, the blood sugar level goes up, and protein turnover and thereby metabolism are activated. In addition, the immune system is impaired which until then was able to carry out its nightly top performance unimpeded. An excessive cortisol release is the nemesis of restful sleep.

Anyone who sleeps too little during the second half of the night, voluntarily or involuntarily, raises his cortisol level considerably until it is so high that the affected person feels distressed. Conversely a high level causes us to sleep badly and to wake up continuously. Poor sleep quality during the first half of the night lets the cortisol level rise substantially, and as a result restful sleep is out of the picture. This is fundamentally important for the regeneration ability or the development of physical performance capacity, especially in competitive athletes.

Important advice

Optimal mattress or sleeping surface quality reduces the release of cortisol. Based on our experiences and stress hormone measurements in saliva, competitive athletes and executives who slept on a viscoelastic material show a markedly improved sleep quality. Competitive athletes take the opportunity to bring a flexible mattress pad in their bag on out-of-town training trips or competitions.

CREATE A RELAXING SLEEP ENVIRONMENT

In fig. 82 we can see that competitive athletes who have slept on the high-tech innovation by Tempur, a pressure-relief mattress developed for NASA's space travel, showed a significantly lower cortisol release the next morning than the competitive athletes who slept on a customary box spring mattress. All competitive athletes (endurance athletes: age distribution: 23.5 ± 4.3) completed the same training during the day until going to sleep.

The 25 executives who slept on the viscoelastic mattress also report subjectively improved sleep quality as compared to the 25 executives who slept on the customary box spring mattresses. Cortisol levels support this unequivocally (see fig. 83).

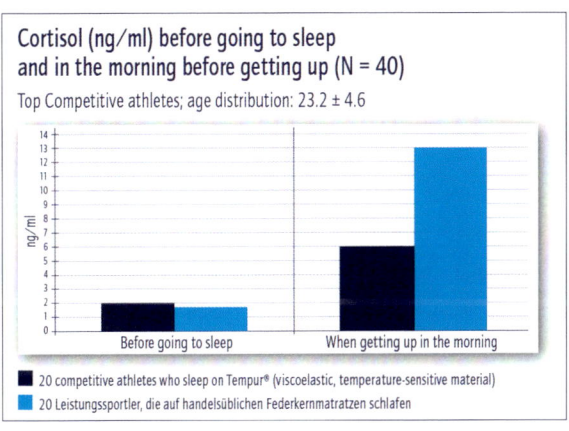

Fig. 82

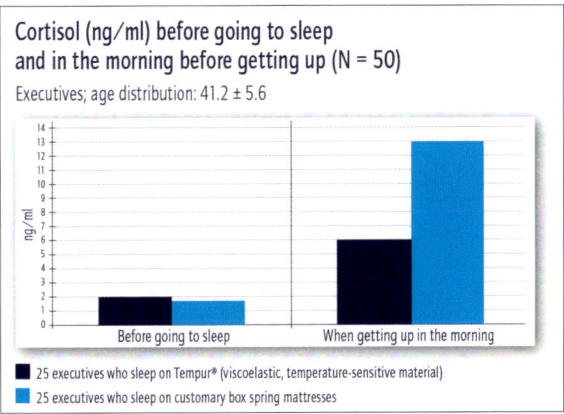

Fig. 83

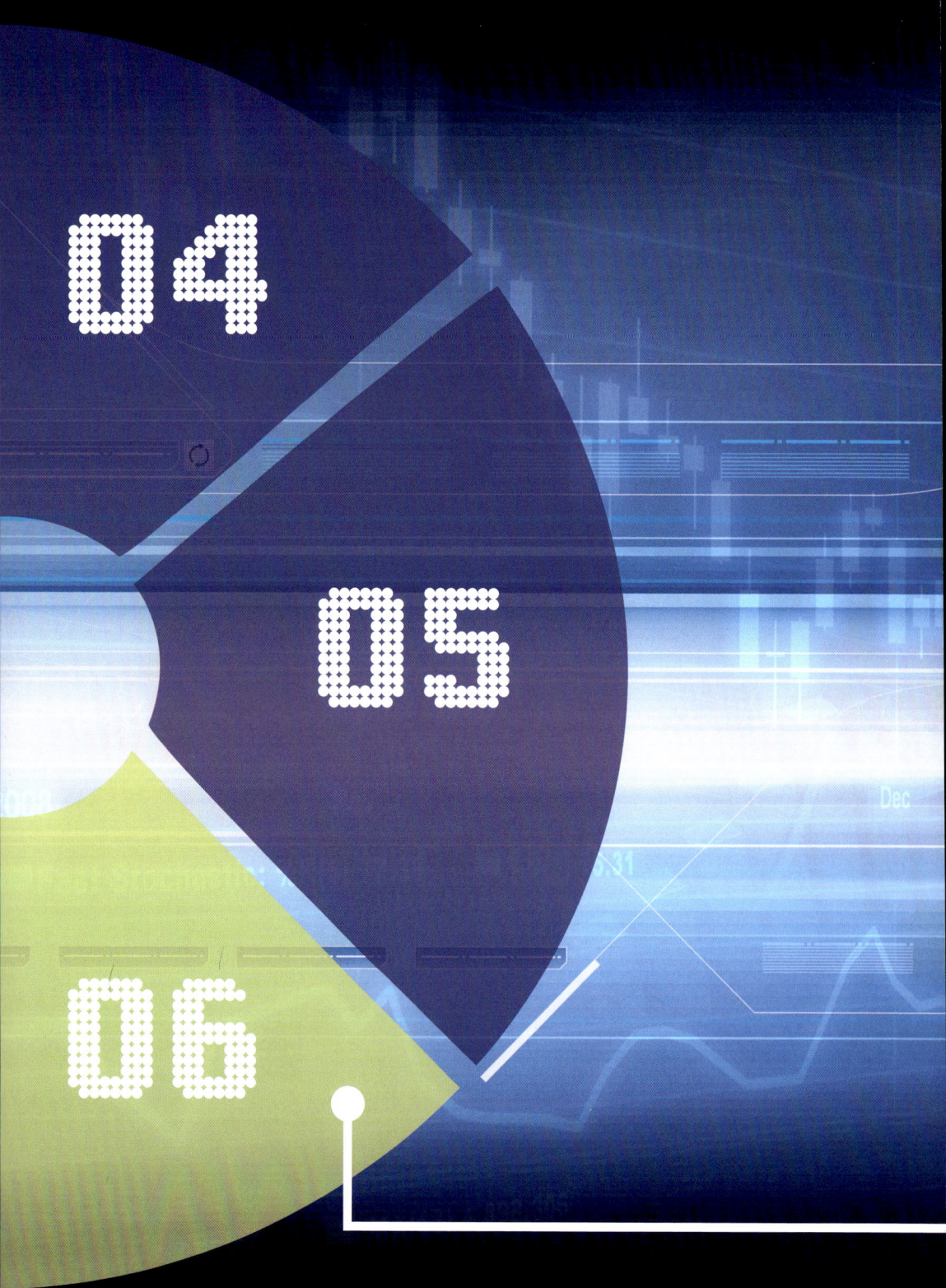

STRESS REDUCTION ON A BIOCHEMICAL LEVEL

6 STRESS REDUCTION ON A BIOCHEMICAL LEVEL

6.1 GENERAL ASPECTS OF CORTISOL

Cortisol controls activity-related and stress reactions. Cortisol is one of the most important hormones overall. It has a highly-developed circadian rhythm. It is produced during the second half of the night, so it is fully available for daytime activities and stresses. It is thus the most important stress hormone that is released during mental or physical stress. It is produced in the adrenal cortex under the brain's influence (hypothalamus) and the pituitary gland (hypophysis). It activates the metabolism, facilitates glucose production, changes the mental reaction status, and interferes greatly with the immune system.

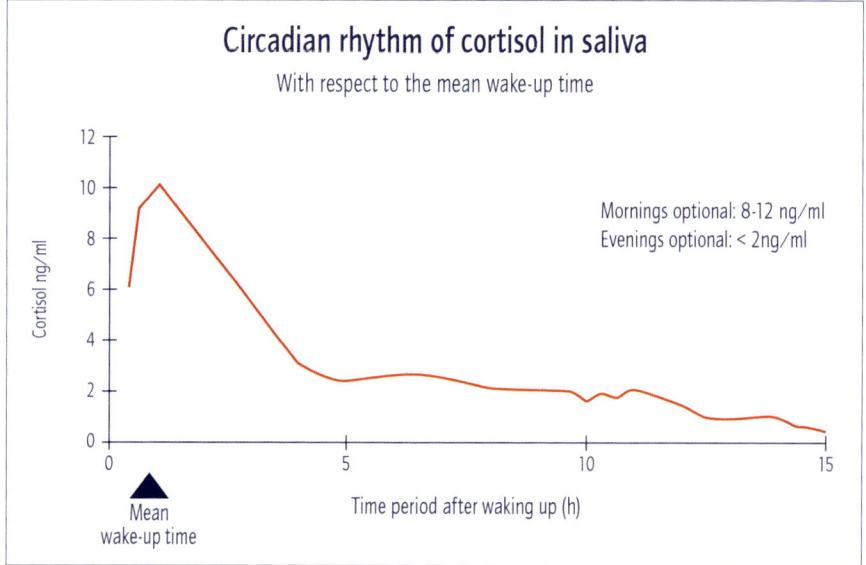

Fig. 84

Unlike adrenaline, cortisol is produced for storage, primarily during the second half of the night, and between 7 and 8 am it is ready for the day's activities and to cope with stress. Cortisol levels drop dramatically in the course of the day, especially midmorning, and at night only 10% of the morning's levels remain. Cortisol is not subject to any appreciable age-specific changes.

Chronically elevated cortisol

Chronically elevated cortisol (reference range: morning > 13 ng/ml, an indicator for hypercortisolism) leads to excess weight, diabetes mellitus, depression, immunodeficiency, and changes to the skin. Elevated cortisol is a result of a malfunction by the hypothalamus and pituitary gland.

Cortisol deficiency

Cortisol deficiency (reference range: morning < 5 ng/ml and during the day < 3ng/ml an indicator for hypocortisolism) leads to lassitude, lack of motivation, infections as well as impairment of immune function. A lack of cortisol can be caused by malfunctions of the adrenal gland, and faulty control of the hypothalamus and the pituitary gland. Cortisol deficiency is also a result of long-term stress and is almost routinely present in cases of chronic fatigue syndrome.

DIURNAL STRESS PROFILE:
INDEPENDENT MEASUREMENT WITH SALIVA SAMPLES

Nowadays measuring cortisol from saliva is a simple and accurate method. Meanwhile cortisol measurements from saliva show a high correlation (0.98) between blood tests and saliva diagnostics.

The normal cortisol level in saliva is subject to dynamic fluctuation. Normal cortisol levels are between 5-15 ng/ml in the morning, while levels in the late afternoon and evening are between 0.3-3 ng/ml. Based on our experience from recent years, a cortisol concentration of < 6 ng/ml in the morning or > 12 ng/ml indicates a very stressed vegetative nervous system. The decisive criterion is the intraindividual variance in tested subjects.

The example of 151 executives (age distribution: 41.3 ± 6.3) shows us what the cortisol sequence looks like (see fig. 85). With 17 ng/ml around 8 am, it is already in a very stressed phase. The test subjects already report a subjective feeling of pressure in the morning, and not being able to power down in a vegetative sense during the day. Around 10 pm these executives are at 8 ng/ml and are unable to sleep all night. From the start, the inadequate energy balance of these executives, as well as the overall view of 4,140 executives, shows various disorders (see chapter 1.3). After three months of an individualized micronutrient formula and substantial change and optimization of the energy balance (see chapter 1.3), the cortisol levels of 151 executives show a definite normalization (fig. 85). They feel considerably better.

Current stress profile analysis

Measurements are taken four times in the course of the day and can provide an optimal illustration of what your current stress sequence looks like:

- 1st test: 8:00 am
- 2nd test: 12:00 pm
- 3rd test: 4:00 pm
- 4th test: 10:00 pm

Send the four saliva samples to SALUTO (web address is in the appendix, pg. 206). A simple method to ascertain your current stress profile.

The cortisol measurements in the form of a diurnal profile show a definite long-term improved stress tolerance. The positive effects of the concept for success "Prescription for Energy" can be seen not only in the special blood and urine analyses but also in the measurements of the stress hormone cortisol.

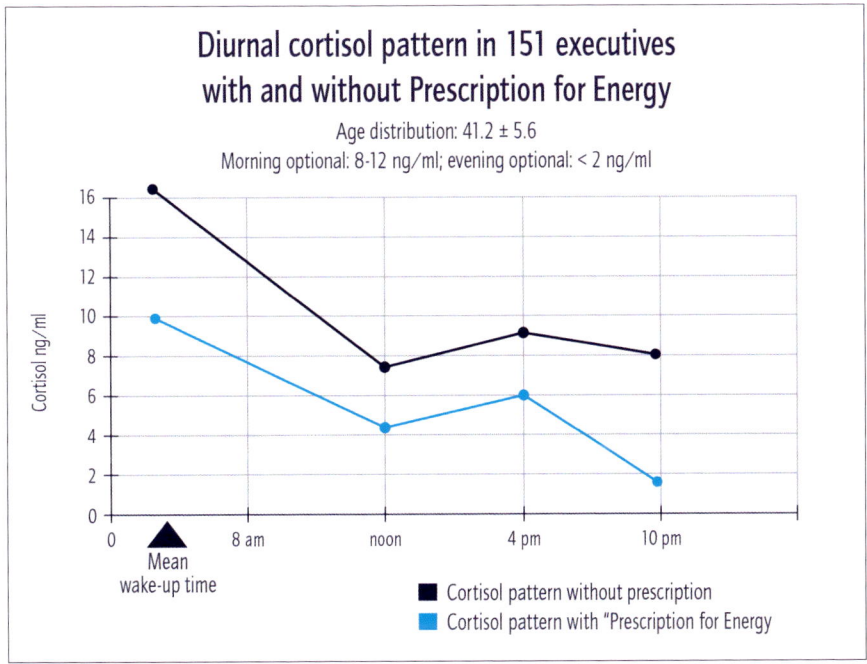

Fig. 85

6.2 SUGAR-RELATED STRESS

Dr. Kurt Mosetter from the Center for Interdisciplinary Therapies has been doing scientific and especially practically-orientated research for years on the many effects of sugar on human performance capacity. He takes care of many internationally successful top athletes in conjunction with the Myoreflex therapy developed by him. Did you know that most people who like to eat sweets at night are subject to extreme stress (i.e., don't sleep as well and regenerate less successfully after athletic exertion)?

The following contribution by Kurt Mosetter offers a simple outline of these interesting facts.

CHRONIC STRESSES AND STRAINS ON THE NEUROBIOCHEMICAL LEVEL

Dr. Kurt Mosetter

Summary

Stress is a phenomenon that is well documented from many perspectives and system levels in scientific treatises (see Fischer, G., Eichenberg, C., Mosetter, K. & Mosetter, R., 2006). Here the focus shall be on the molecular synaptic network level (see Mosetter, K., 2008 and also Reutter, W. & Mosetter, K., 2006).

Stress (distress) and its physiological functions are meant to make the organism of the person experiencing it maximally efficient under short-term mobilization of all physical resources during an emergency, in dangerous situations, vital challenges, danger in battle, or during flight from danger. Stress reactions become abnormal only under chronic stress with long-term dysregulation of homeostasis. Unlike animals, who usually only experience or require short-term stress activations, humans deal with constant stress (see Sapolsky, R. M., 1995). This does not only throw off physical regulation in terms of hypertension, higher heart rate, diabetogenic state of the metabolism, and the respective stress hormones with cortisol, adrenaline, and noradrenaline, and also neurobiochemical circuits.

Stress management on the cellular level
Stress and constant strain have many faces and are subject to nearly endless trigger situations. The most basic stress management takes place in our cells. A healthy stress response, the mastering and modulation of all the steps, depend on cellular communication. These steps also control preventative processes and associated repairs after extreme stress situations. Ordinarily our organism is perfectly prepared for and adapted to stress related to its growth, development, and aging. But long-term stress leads to problems and requires unusual amounts of energy while simultaneously adjusting normal performances and basic functions.

Organic elements and sugar structures are vitally important in several ways to ensure these steps. Chronic stress and distress are evident on the cellular level, particularly by an increased sugar consumption of the brain. To maintain the vital "frontline functions" (energy metabolism), and "second line functions" (anabolism to maintain the structural integrity of cells and organs) are permanently neglected.

Figuratively speaking, we can imagine it this way: During a cold winter we need wood for heating so we don't freeze to death. But then we don't have the wood to repair defective windows, doors, or roofs. When this state persists for too long or repeats itself each year, the house begins to deteriorate or becomes irreparable. We might not freeze, or may be we are a little cold, but the house falls down. It is similar with the sugar structures that now can only be used for energy production, but are barely available to maintain the integrity of the brain cells.

During a stress reaction, all daily processes such as digestion, immune system, and nerve cell growth clearly take the backseat. Flight-or-fight survival strategies increasingly come to the forefront. But long-term suppression of the usual functions, which are designed and perfected for short-term stresses, leads to states that severely affect health. Increased susceptibility to illness, infections, and cardiovascular diseases can also result from this.

The significance of stress disorder and stress prevention also becomes obvious here, as well as the need to supply the body with all necessary substances for stress management, repair, buffering, and even prevention. The basic structures for all these steps are simple sugars.

Blood sugar and stress
There is a close correlation between blood sugar and stress. During extreme stress the organism prepares to overcome a threat by flight or fight behavior. This requires primarily energy and an appropriate blood sugar level. During stress, the blood sugar metabolism works according to an emergency plan. To do so, sugar reserves are released from the liver into the blood. In addition, the pulse rate and blood pressure go up. In contrast, normal and resting functions such as digestion are reduced.

Stress is typically linked with a rise in cortisol and CRH (corticotropin releasing hormone). Corticosteroids and insulin behave antagonistically. Increased cortisol effects result in altered insulin effects. Blood sugar levels remain higher during the physiological readiness action (phylogenetic for flight, threat, fight in terms of crucial survival). When chronic—constant stress—these conditions lead to insulin resistance. Insulin resistance and impaired insulin signal transduction lead to impaired glucose utilization and a state of cellular energy deficiency. The cells are receiving too little glucose. This reduces the availability of important neurotransmitters (GABA, acetylcholine, glycine, glutamate).

The sugar metabolism and its derailment thus play a major role in stress-related conditions and illnesses.

A lack of energy develops via ammonia (NH3) in the stress metabolism and under constant stress. Ammonia is toxic and also has a performance-inhibiting effect (see Schulz, H. & Heck, H., 2006).

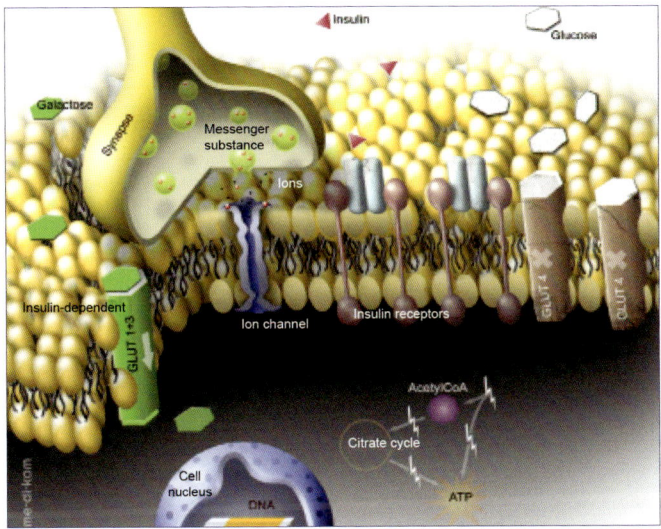

Fig. 86

The energy metabolism equation

Oxidative stress: The greater the physical or psycho-mental stresses, the more chronic stress reproduces as oxidative stress (with harmful free radicals) in the organism. A number of the body's own defensive systems helps to intercept and reduce the number of free radicals (OH, O_2, OONO-). Vitamin C, Vitamin E, melatonin, coenzyme Q_{10}, and secondary plant substances such as OPC support the antioxidative defense. At the same time the source of free radicals (O_2, uric acid, and ammonia) should be strengthened from the root, meaning from a stressed (weak) energy metabolism equation, in such a way that the many free radials cannot even form, and the work of the energy power stations, the cells (mitochondria), is activated.

Two natural and smart simple sugars—galactose and ribose—are able to achieve antioxidative and energy metabolism-stabilizing spectrum efficacy on multiple levels.

Galactose:
- Absorption is insulin-independent.
- Improves availability of glucose inside cells.
- Balances metabolic stress-related glucose deficiency.
- Ensures endogenous detoxification (binding and removal of ammonia) and ensures recycling (metabolization) to amino acids.
- Has a synthesizing anabolic effect (enhanced protein synthesis).
- Has an extended performance profile; helps the organism remain in an economical, anaerobic metabolism for an extended period of time.
- Ensures the integration of glycogen, especially in the muscles.
- Ensures a balanced anabolic metabolism.

Ribose:
- Strengthens the energy metabolism.
- Is the "sugar" for the energy power stations in the cells, the mitochondria.
- Is the basic structure for our genes, DNA, and RNA.
- Improves cardiac function.
- Improves brain metabolism.
- Improves muscle metabolism.
- Improves training performance.
- Improves mitochondrial function.
- Improves regeneration metabolism.
- Is a basic element of the ultimate carrier of energy, ATP.
- As a five-membered ring sugar it does not raise the blood sugar level.
- Is a monosaccharide and therefore does not have to be cleaved in the intestines.
- Has a strong antioxidant effect
- Is the "Espresso substitute."

Since the organism's absorption of the monosaccharide galactose is insulin independent, this simple and natural sugar substance can sidestep the cellular supply crunch via a molecular bypass. Galcatose reaches the cell, picks up NH_3 equivalents, synthesizes amino acids, and ensures the energy balance as well as the anabolic metabolism for neurotransmitters and cell membrane.

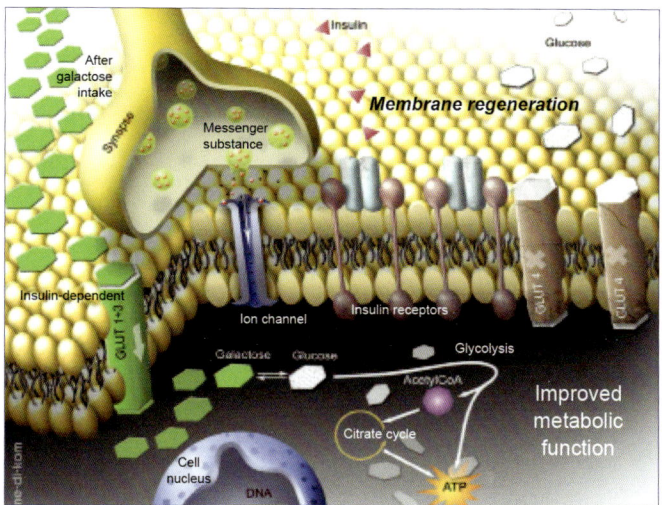

Fig. 87

The sugar structure galactose is important for the forming, structure, and function of vital glycoproteins and glycolipids. This substance ensures the stabilization of the cell surface, and cell-to-cell communication and recognition. It thereby increases concentration, memory, alertness, action, and decision-making ability.

Ribose is another important and helpful sugar structure. Lack of energy and mitochondrial dysfunction are the forces behind many neurovegetative problems: fatigue, lack of motivation, weakness, weak or lacking immune response, anxiety, retention and memory problems, movement disorders, and muscle tension.

Here ribose can serve as the sugar for the cells' energy power stations, the mitochondria (see Addis, P., Shecterle, L. M., & Alexander, J., 2012, as well as: Teitelbaum, J. E., 2007, Teitelbaum, J. E., Johnson, C. & St. Cyr, J., 2006). It improves mitochondrial function and thereby cardiac function, brain metabolism, muscle metabolism, as well as regeneration metabolism. Ribose is the basic element for the ultimate carrier of energy ATP and as a five-ring sugar does not raise the blood sugar level. As a monosaccharide (simple sugar), it does not have to be cleaved in the intestines. In addition, ribose has a strong antioxidant effect (see Mostetter, K., Pape, D. & Cavelius, A., 2002, as well as Mosetter, K. & Reutter, W., 2007, Roser, M., Josic, D., Kontou, M., Mosetter, K., Maurer, P. & Reutter, W., 2009).

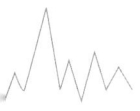

No rest at night—no energy during the day

Often sleep is disrupted by work-related stress and constant tension. This can quickly turn into a viscous cycle: lack of sleep and disrupted sleep facilitate insulin resistance (see Schmid, S. M., Hallschmid, M., Jauch-Chara, K., Wilms, B., Lehnert, H., Born, J. & Schultes, B., 2011), which in turn often results in increased consumption of carbohydrates and thus continued cellular stress.

Our daily routine is shaped by internal rhythms that characterize our activity and performance spectrums. Depending on the metabolic state, melatonin is synthesized from serotonin. These syntheses depend on light irradiation, stress level, cortisol and insulin metabolism, and regulated enzymatic activity.

In cases of stress-associated rhythm abnormalities there is often a lack of cortisol release in the mornings, the trigger for physiological activity. In contrast, relatively high cortisol levels in the evening and at night lead to restlessness, insomnia, and inability to relax during those times. At the same time cortisol activity during periods of rest lead to compensatory calming attempts, often via excessive consumption of sweets. When a lot of cortisol is released in the evening, serotonin and melatonin become less active during the night. This internal lack of calmness causes a shift in the sleep rhythm. Resting activity develops in the morning and throughout the day; difficulty getting started, lack of motivation, fatigue, and lassitude characterize the morning hours and the course of the day.

A critical external stimulus for melatonin production is daylight. But new research findings show that except for light, all of the body's information—and particularly the upper cervical spine on the way to the pineal gland (epiphysis), the place where melatonin is produced—participates in determining rhythm.

Neuroanatomically the pineal gland is not directly activated, but rather receives stimuli to activate melatonin production indirectly, via a detour and interconnections in the upper cervical spine (see Mosetter, K. & Mosetter, R., 2010, as well as Mosetter, K. & Mosetter, R., 2008).

STRESS REDUCTION ON A BIOCHEMICAL LEVEL

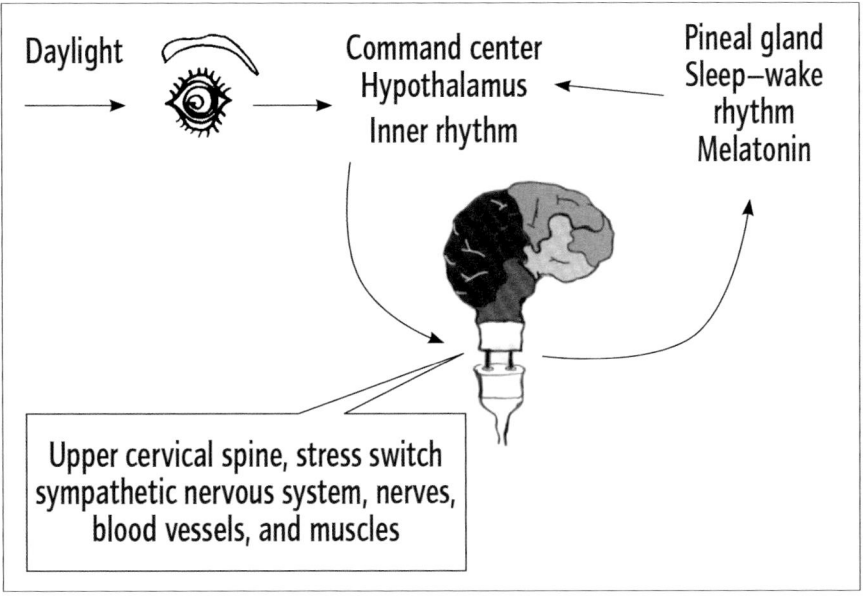

Fig. 88

Major tension and malposition of the upper cervical spine cause irritation of the melatonin pathway and thereby disruption of the sleep–wake rhythm and internal clock. Conversely, neuromuscular regulation of these regions can be achieved via myoreflex therapy. Furthermore, specific physical exercises can bring considerable relief (see Mosetter, K. & Mosetter, R. as well as Mosetter, K. & Mosetter, R., 2008).

6.3 PREVENTION WITH PRESCRIPTION FOR ENERGY

Results from comprehensive testing, the early detection and correction of biochemical disorders, is one of the main tasks in the prevention of exhaustion. Our experience with the executives who were tested show 100% compliance with the use of the Prescription for Energy concept. With the use of this concept verifiable states of exhaustion (The battery is dead on all levels. The feeling that you can't go on because you feel weak, unmotivated, and unhappy) can be prevented.

Of the executives we tested, as well as 6,120 other employees, 70% were dissatisfied with their diets but claim that they are unable to make significant changes. There were other factors along with nutritional deficiencies (see chapter 5.2).

The results presented previously might give the impression that executives (entrepreneurs, executive managers, executive staff) depend on a continued targeted intake of micronutrients, and that a good diet has a much lesser effect on the micronutrient balance than previously thought. But far from it! It is true that there is an urgent need for a targeted, individualized micronutrient formula (not based on the shotgun approach and the belief that "more helps more"). Anyone who thinks he can ease his guilty conscience with a regular intake of vitamins, minerals, and trace elements according to the motto "eat fast food and pop pills" has not understood the problem. Combining both is fundamentally important (see pg. 76-77).

An optimal balance of biochemical processes verifiably leads to vitality, quality of life, and increased performance capacity (see chapter 4, Biochemistry of happiness). With the use of the "Prescription for Energy" concept and the correction of initially-detected biochemical disorders, definite improvements in the delineated disorders can be seen within just a few months (see pg. 22, fig. 4, and pg. 23, fig. 5).

Energy balance status quo

Of 4,150 executives (entrepreneurs, executive managers, and executive staff) and 6,120 employees; age distribution: 44.3 ± 9.2

Beginning | After 3 months of Prescription for Energy

Functional energy metabolism

	Beginning	After 3 months
Citric acid	insufficient	borderline
Cis-aconitic acid	insufficient	good
Alpha-ketoglutaric acid	insufficient	good
Succinic acid	insufficient	good
Fumaric acid	good	good
Malic acid	good	good

Amino acids

	Beginning	After 3 months
Preservation of connective tissue structure function	insufficient	good
Neurotransmitter activity	borderline	borderline
Stabilization of energy balance (BCAAs)	insufficient	good
Brain metabolism	insufficient	borderline

Micronutrient concentration

	Beginning	After 3 months
Magnesium	insufficient	good
Zinc	insufficient	borderline
Selenium	insufficient	good
Vitamin B_1	insufficient	borderline
Vitamin B_2	insufficient	good
Vitamin B_6	insufficient	good
Vitamin B_9	insufficient	good
Vitamin B_{12}	insufficient	good

Demand on the body's own structural proteins

	Beginning	After 3 months
Cartilage (PD)	borderline	borderline
Bone (DPD)	borderline	borderline

Initial disorders

- Light night sweats
- Restless sleep
- Agitation
- Poor stress tolerance (quick loss of composure)
- Increasing fatigue, some lack of motivation
- Combined with some difficulty concentrating
- Muscle tension
- Trouble unwinding after work
- Increasing personal stress

After 3 months of Prescription for Energy

- No more night sweats
- Restful sleep
- Even temper
- Good stress tolerance (composure in stressful situations)
- Creative and not tired
- Good concentration ability
- Able to unwind after work
- Even temper in personal life

Key: very good | good | borderline | insufficient

Fig. 89

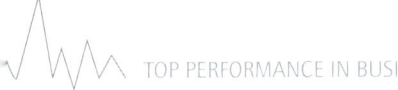

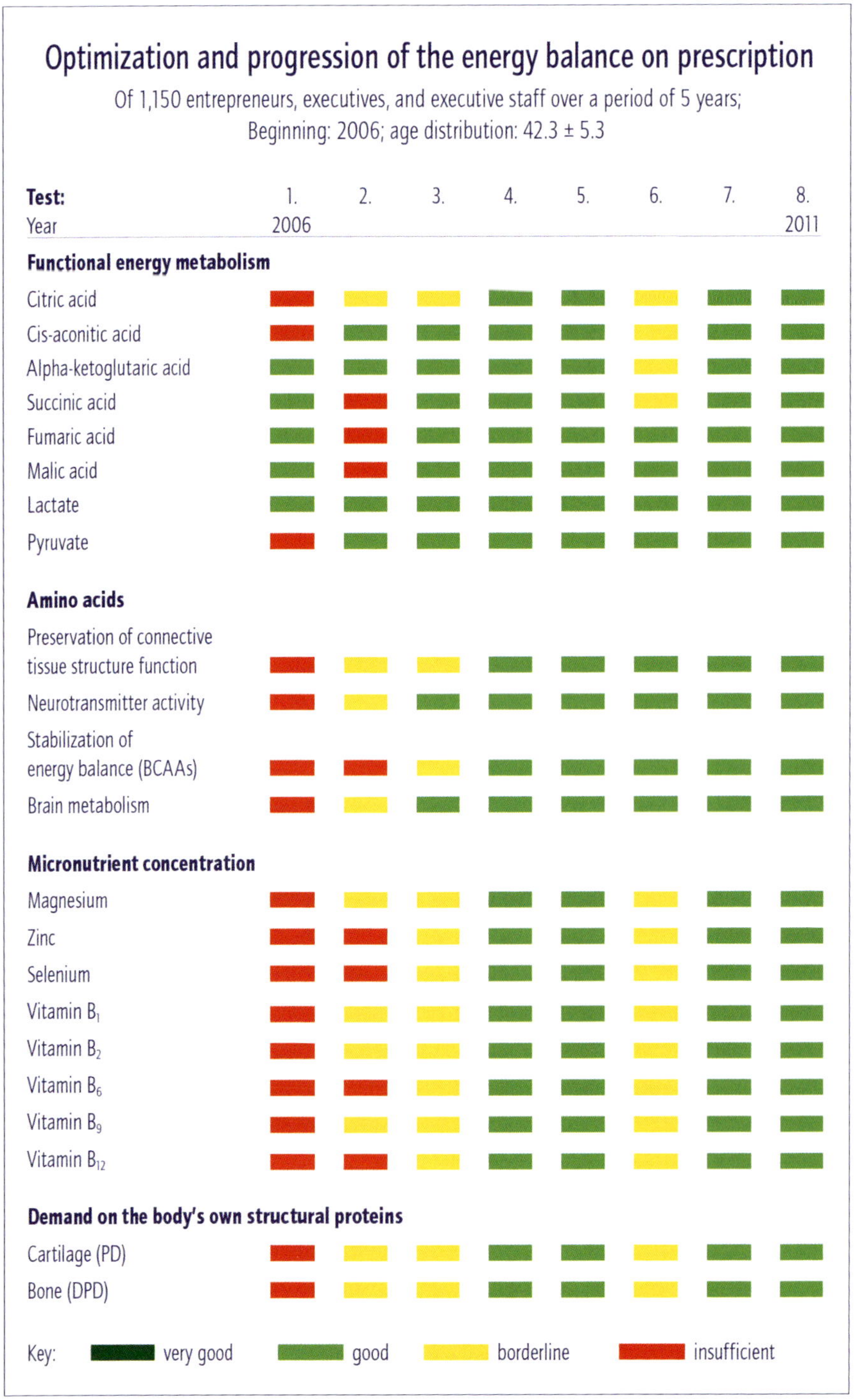

Optimization and progression of the energy balance on prescription

Of 1,150 entrepreneurs, executives, and executive staff over a period of 5 years;
Beginning: 2006; age distribution: 42.3 ± 5.3

Test: Year	1. 2006	2.	3.	4.	5.	6.	7.	8. 2011
Functional energy metabolism								
Citric acid	insufficient	borderline	borderline	very good	very good	borderline	very good	very good
Cis-aconitic acid	insufficient	good	very good	very good	very good	borderline	very good	very good
Alpha-ketoglutaric acid	good	very good	very good	very good	borderline	very good	very good	very good
Succinic acid	good	insufficient	very good	very good	very good	very good	very good	very good
Fumaric acid	good	good	insufficient	very good	very good	very good	very good	very good
Malic acid	good	good	insufficient	very good	very good	very good	very good	very good
Lactate	good	good	good	very good	very good	very good	very good	very good
Pyruvate	insufficient	good	good	very good	very good	very good	very good	very good
Amino acids								
Preservation of connective tissue structure function	insufficient	borderline	borderline	very good	very good	very good	very good	very good
Neurotransmitter activity	insufficient	borderline	good	very good	very good	very good	very good	very good
Stabilization of energy balance (BCAAs)	insufficient	borderline	borderline	very good	very good	very good	very good	very good
Brain metabolism	insufficient	borderline	good	very good	very good	very good	very good	very good
Micronutrient concentration								
Magnesium	insufficient	borderline	borderline	very good	very good	borderline	very good	very good
Zinc	insufficient	insufficient	borderline	very good	very good	very good	very good	very good
Selenium	insufficient	insufficient	borderline	very good	very good	very good	very good	very good
Vitamin B_1	insufficient	borderline	borderline	very good	very good	very good	very good	very good
Vitamin B_2	insufficient	borderline	borderline	very good	very good	very good	very good	very good
Vitamin B_6	insufficient	insufficient	borderline	very good	very good	very good	very good	very good
Vitamin B_9	insufficient	borderline	borderline	very good	very good	very good	very good	very good
Vitamin B_{12}	insufficient	insufficient	borderline	very good	very good	very good	very good	very good
Demand on the body's own structural proteins								
Cartilage (PD)	insufficient	borderline	borderline	very good	very good	very good	very good	very good
Bone (DPD)	insufficient	borderline	borderline	borderline	very good	very good	very good	very good

Key: very good | good | borderline | insufficient

Fig. 90

STRESS REDUCTION ON A BIOCHEMICAL LEVEL

Optimization and progression of the energy balance in 1,150 entrepreneurs, executives, and executive staff over the period of six years (time period 2006-2011, see fig. 90) with an optimal prescription energy intake shows how the initial deficiencies normalize over the following years.

The different energy metabolism measurements were done twice a year with the appropriate adjustment to the personal prescription. You can refer to the example cases (see chapters 7.2 and 7.3) to see the various components of this prescription.

The self-report by 1,150 executives (see fig. 92) shows how the Prescription for Energy concept subjectively impacted performance capacity. In just a short period of time the individualized prescription energy intake brought about fantastic results with respect to the delineated disorders. Detection (special analysis) and correction of biochemical disorders always brought the desired results. That is why we refer to the Biochemistry of happiness. Human energy requirement depends on lifestyle, potential prior illnesses, and physical/professional activity. The self-report by 1,150 executives (see fig. 92) shows how the Prescription for Energy concept had a subjective effect on performance capacity.

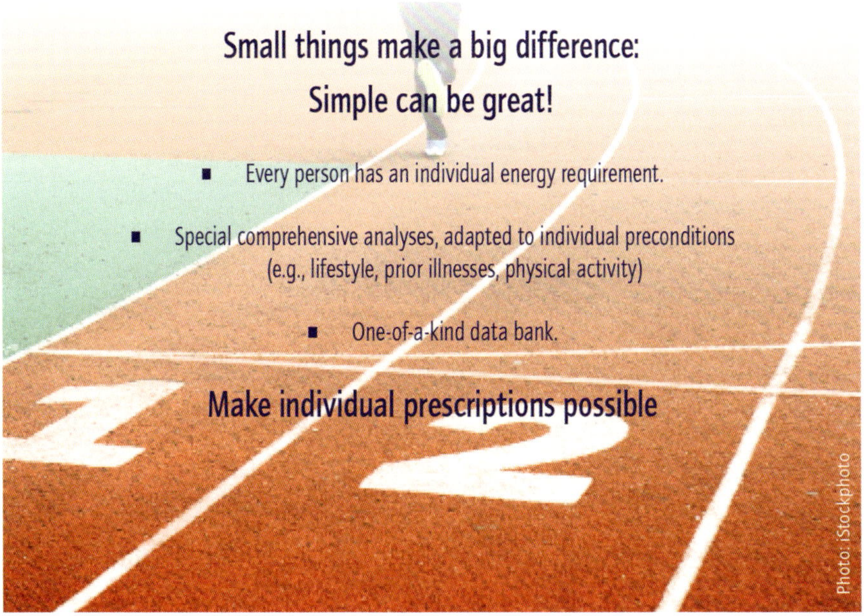

Small things make a big difference: Simple can be great!

- Every person has an individual energy requirement.
- Special comprehensive analyses, adapted to individual preconditions (e.g., lifestyle, prior illnesses, physical activity)
- One-of-a-kind data bank.

Make individual prescriptions possible

Fig. 91

> **Self-report by 1,150 entrepreneurs, executives, and executive staff over a period of 6 years after a prescription energy and micronutrient intake.**
>
> At first we were very skeptical, but after only six weeks we already noticed:
>
> - No more night sweats
> - Considerably improved sleep pattern
> - Better stress tolerance (improved composure during stress phases)
> - Clearly better mood
> - Improved mental and physical ability to withstand stress
> - Verifiably improved our immune system and reduced infection rate
> - Subjective feeling of improved mental and physical performance capacity
> - Prescription for Energy has become our gold standard
> - There is verifiably no better system that will guarantee long-term well-being and creativity over a 6-year time period while daily stress actually increases

Abb. 92

6.4 COMPETITVE AND ELITE SPORTS WITH PRESCRIPTION FOR ENERGY: THE PROVEN RECIPE FOR TRAINING CONTINUITY AND TOP PERFORMANCE

Top performances are only possible when the athlete is healthy and is able to tap his full performance potential without training interruptions. Early detection and correction of biochemical disorders is one of the main aspects in competitive and elite sports. Of the 11,150 top competitive athletes tested by SALUTO, 70% reported increasing exhaustion and major performance fluctuations. Of these athletes, 71% exhibited *no-contact injuries* resulting from overloading reactions (for additional information see chapter 1.4). In the beginning, the comprehensive analyses show severe activity impairments of certain enzymes in the energy metabolism, which resulted in biochemical disorders with various ailments. Our studies are corroborated by an anonymous survey by the Cologne Sports College on behalf of the German Sports Aid Foundation (see fig. 13, pg. 32).

Increasing mental and physical demands can only be tolerated when the athletes have an optimal energy status. But this requires an appropriately comprehensive analysis (see chapter 1.4) that isn't performed in the field. Especially the timely detection of excessive demand on the body's own structural proteins can help stabilize the athlete's performance potential long-term.

With individualized Prescription for Energy the many biochemical disorders we detected in the 11,150 top competitive athletes can be considerably decreased after only six months, although there is continued potential for optimization (see fig. 15, pg. 34). The positive change in the energy balance shows definite correlations between optimal energy balance and an athlete's performance capacity; 100% describe a direct link between "Prescription for Energy" and athletic success.

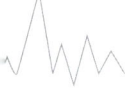
TOP PERFORMANCE IN BUSINESS AND SPORTS

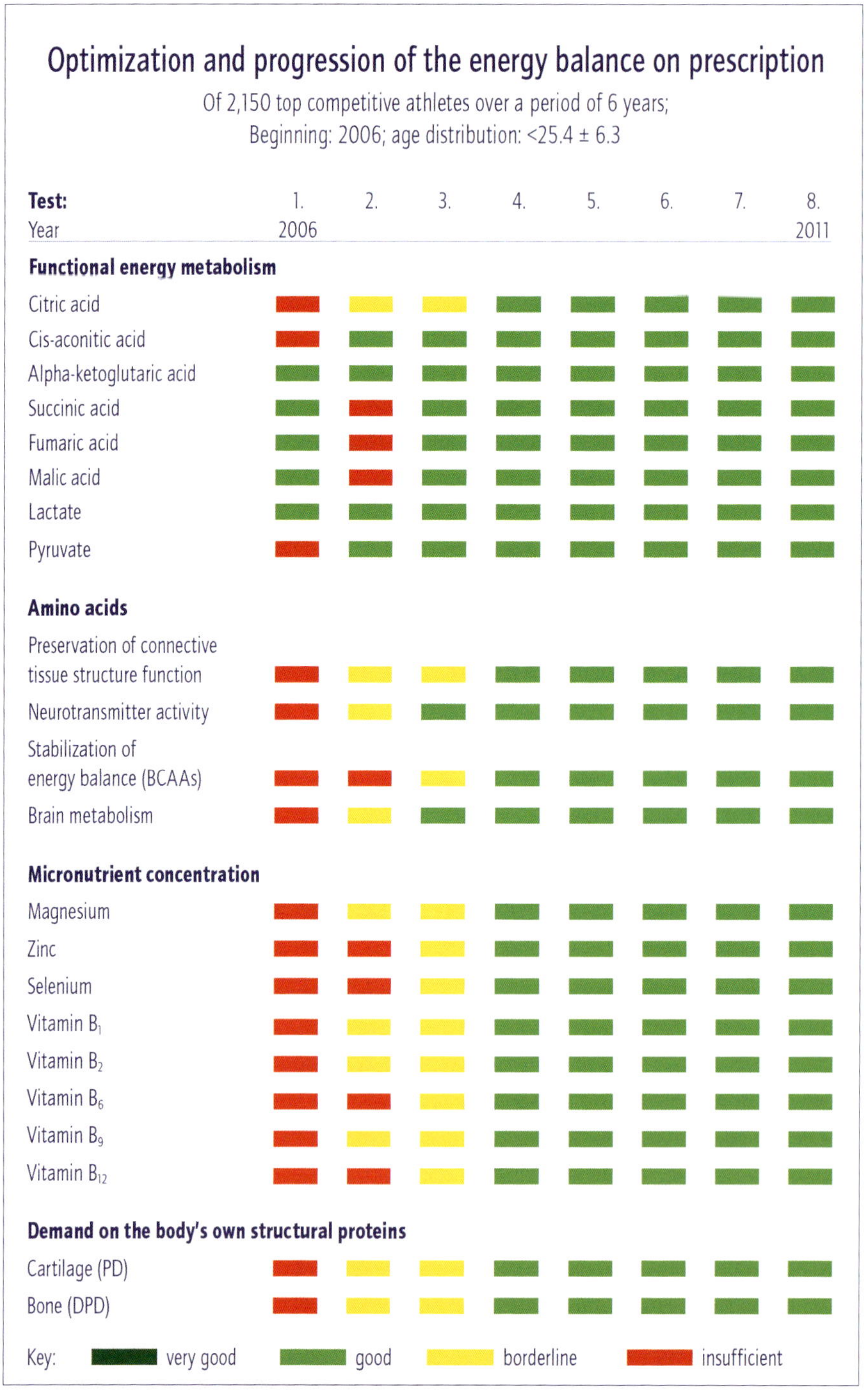

Optimization and progression of the energy balance on prescription

Of 2,150 top competitive athletes over a period of 6 years;
Beginning: 2006; age distribution: <25.4 ± 6.3

Test: Year	1. 2006	2.	3.	4.	5.	6.	7.	8. 2011
Functional energy metabolism								
Citric acid	insufficient	borderline	borderline	good	good	good	good	good
Cis-aconitic acid	insufficient	good	good	good	good	good	good	good
Alpha-ketoglutaric acid	good	good	good	good	good	good	good	good
Succinic acid	good	insufficient	good	good	good	good	good	good
Fumaric acid	good	insufficient	insufficient	good	good	good	good	good
Malic acid	good	insufficient	insufficient	good	good	good	good	good
Lactate	good	good	good	good	good	good	good	good
Pyruvate	insufficient	good	good	good	good	good	good	good
Amino acids								
Preservation of connective tissue structure function	insufficient	borderline	borderline	good	good	good	good	good
Neurotransmitter activity	insufficient	borderline	good	good	good	good	good	good
Stabilization of energy balance (BCAAs)	insufficient	insufficient	borderline	good	good	good	good	good
Brain metabolism	insufficient	good	borderline	good	good	good	good	good
Micronutrient concentration								
Magnesium	insufficient	borderline	borderline	good	good	good	good	good
Zinc	insufficient	insufficient	insufficient	good	good	good	good	good
Selenium	insufficient	insufficient	borderline	good	good	good	good	good
Vitamin B_1	insufficient	borderline	borderline	good	good	good	good	good
Vitamin B_2	insufficient	borderline	borderline	good	good	good	good	good
Vitamin B_6	insufficient	borderline	borderline	good	good	good	good	good
Vitamin B_9	insufficient	borderline	borderline	good	good	good	good	good
Vitamin B_{12}	insufficient	borderline	borderline	good	good	good	good	good
Demand on the body's own structural proteins								
Cartilage (PD)	insufficient	borderline	borderline	good	good	good	good	good
Bone (DPD)	insufficient	borderline	borderline	good	good	good	good	good

Key: ▬ very good ▬ good ▬ borderline ▬ insufficient

Fig. 93

Optimization and progression of the energy balance over a period of six years (time period from 2006-2011, see fig. 93) of 2,150 top competitive athletes with "Prescription for Energy" shows how initial deficiencies normalize over the following years.

The energy metabolism measurements were taken four times a year with appropriate adjustment to the formula. For additional information, you can refer to the example cases (see chapter 7.3) where you can also find the various components of this formula. Many international top athletes (Olympic champions, world, European, and German champions) have benefitted from Prescription for Energy for many years and are thereby able to train intensively at a higher level and tap their full performance potential.

PRESCRIPTION FOR ENERGY INCREASES CONNECTIVE TISSUE ELASTICITY

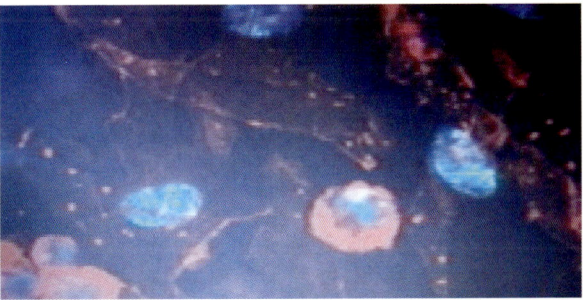

Fig. 94

Initial preliminary examinations show that Prescription for Energy can considerably improve elasticity of stressed connective tissue structures (ligaments, tendons, muscles). This is the case particularly with respect to prevention, but also for athletes who are already injured and are undergoing special rehabilitation. New research shows that increasing quantities of specific protein structures can clearly improve the elasticity of, for instance, ligament structures (see pg. 100-102). Prof. Dr. Helene Langewine, neurologist at the University of Vermont, and her research team have been able to show that a large quantity of these specific protein structures is characteristic for good connective tissue elasticity (see fig. 94). Future research projects will show the verifiable impact of "Prescription for Energy" on these structures.

The self-report of 2,150 top competitive athletes over a six-year time period verifiably documents the positive changes in the energy status (fig. 95) on the subjective sense of well-being of the individual athletes.

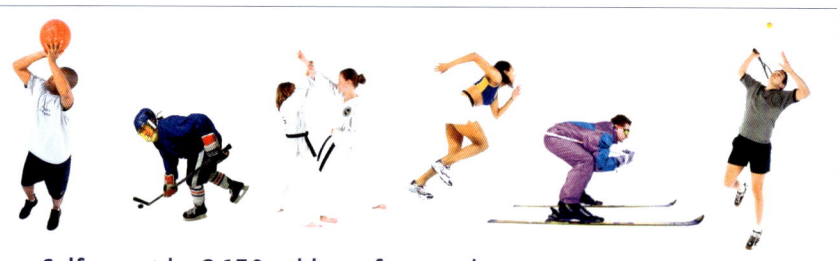

Fig. 95

STRESS REDUCTION ON A BIOCHEMICAL LEVEL

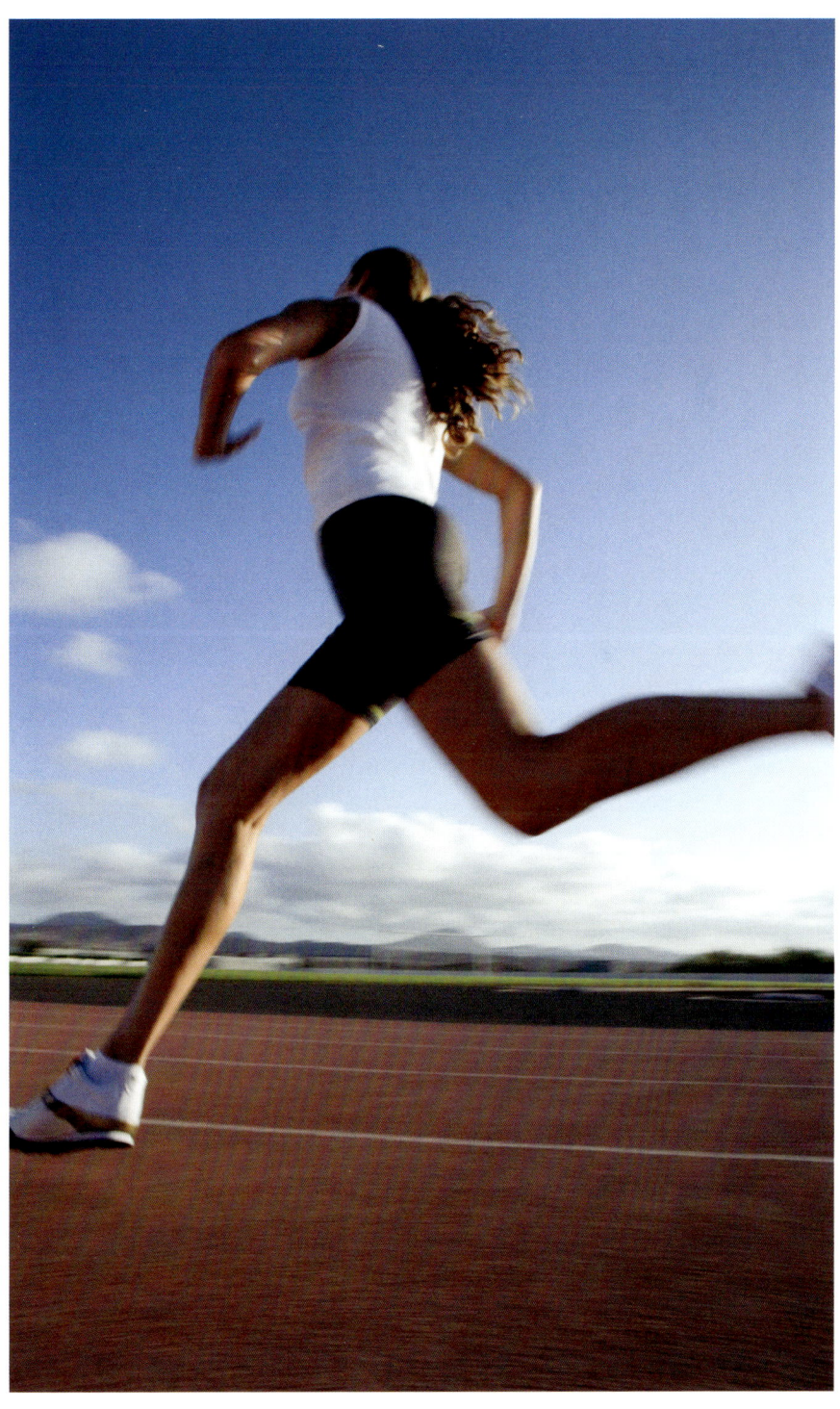

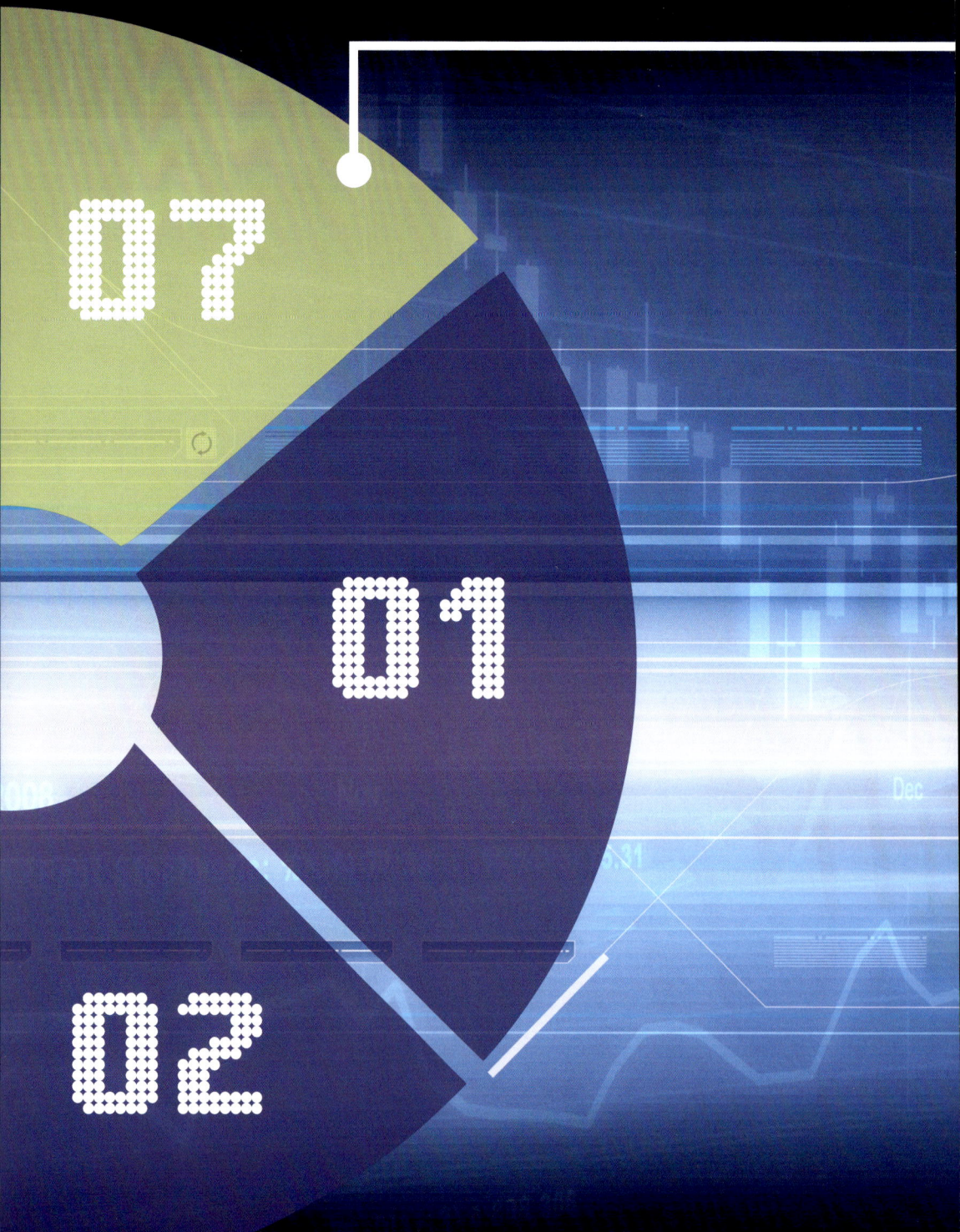

ANALYSIS AND REGULATION

7 ANALYSIS AND REGULATION

7.1 PRESCRIPTION FOR ENERGY: WHAT IS THE PRACTICAL APPPLICATION?

Previous preventative concepts for the preservation of personal well-being are based on a balance of biochemical processes. Optimal "Prescription for Energy", individualized and successful, is based on early detection and correction of biochemical disorders. Different groups of people (executives, and top competitive athletes) whose test results are > 25% of the respective ascertained mean values of the individual micronutrients, show psychophysical stability, no exhaustion, and feel even-tempered and resilient. Assessment of the comprehensive analyses is done in relation to the group of people, age, sex, respective disorders, physical activity, and based on a worldwide comprehensive data bank. For top competitive athletes, the type of sport and the respective timing of training and competition phases are needed to determine the prescription. Balanced thyroid hormones are also very important for vitality and strength (see chapter 2.5). They are therefore taken into account during the preparation of the overall formulas.

VITAL SUBSTANCES IN A BUILDING-BLOCK SYSTEM

The unique building block system of HCK vital nutrient blends is considered a basic supply for an adequate micronutrient concentration that a pharmacist can prepare based on individual prescription. Each individual receives exact dosage specifications. When needed, it is also possible to add arginine, an important amino acid. What makes this system distinctive is the individualized formula that can be adjusted after regular checks of current facts and conditions.

Next to the basic HCK supply, the overall formula can also contain some mono-preparations as needed. These could be magnesium, L-tryptophan, omega-3 fatty acids, Jodid 100, or thyroid medications like L-Thyroxine and iron supplements, but that must be taken separately. This is supplemented with a high-quality amino acid blend. Critical here is not the total amount of protein but the quality of, for instance, the collagen peptides (arginine, methionine, proline) that are fundamentally important for the preservation of stressed connective tissue function (tendons, ligaments, muscles, cartilage).

The balanced composition and bioavailability in the body are critical to the effectiveness of the vital nutrient preparation. The body is best able to absorb vital nutrients that are integrated into plant cells, such as in fruit or vegetables. This is called a *colloidal* state. Anything that grows and serves as a food is in a colloidal state.

HCK® granular micronutrients are vitamins, minerals, trace elements, bioflavonoids, and dietary fiber that are integrated into a plant-based *hydrocolloid* (Guarin, obtained from guar). The resulting resorption properties of the vital nutrients are optimally adapted to each other as they would be in nature. The vital nutrients integrated with the HCK® system:

- ensure optimal distribution in the body;
- ensure delayed release for hours from the gastrointestinal tract;
- prevent disturbance reactions between the vital nutrients;

- are individually adaptable to the respective micronutrient requirements based on functional metabolism results and intracellular micronutrient analysis; and
- combine vitamins, minerals, trace elements, bioflavonoids, and dietary fiber.

Prescription for Energy can verifiably increase the elasticity of stressed connective tissue structures (ligaments, tendons, muscles), has a preventative effect, and in the future will be of outstanding importance for rehabilitation (see pg. 16-17).

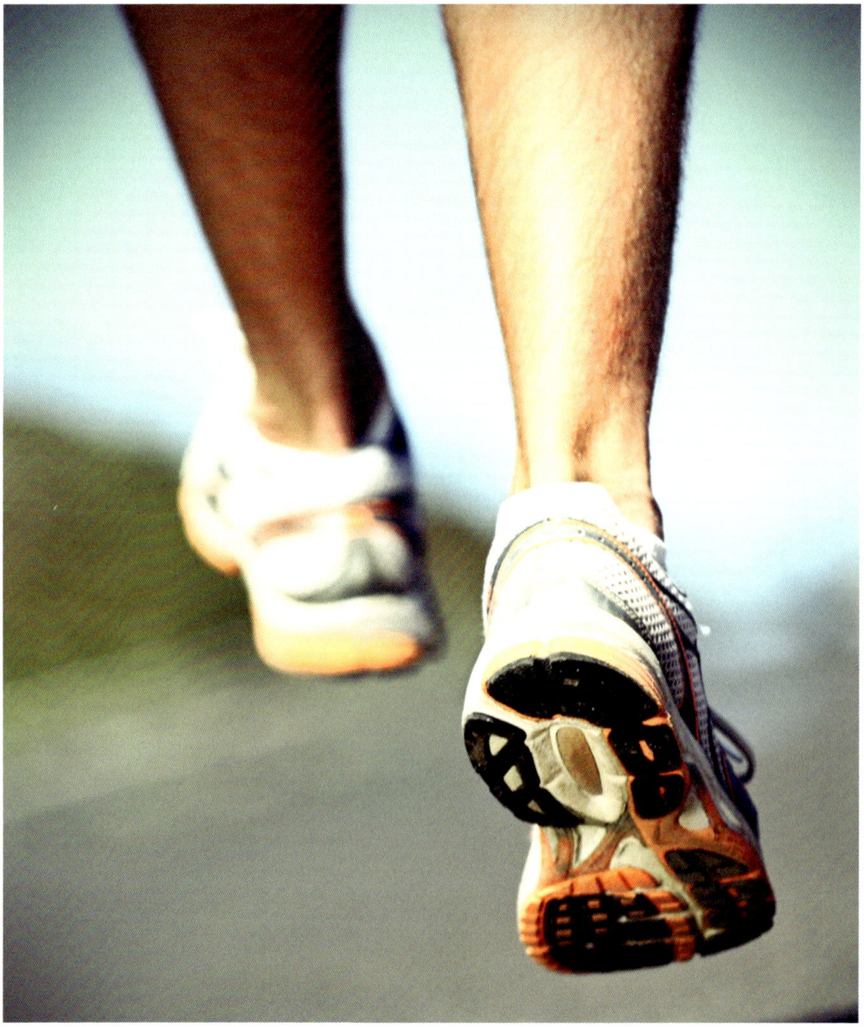

7.2 CASE STUDIES OF EXECUTIVES

EXAMPLE CASE OF A 48-YEAR-OLD EXECUTIVE

The completed anamnesis resulted in the following clinical presentation:

- Board member and HR manager of a computer company with 2,500 associates, divorced, 2 children
- Height: 5'3"
- Weight: 125.6 lbs
- Jogs 1 hour 4x per week (with heart rate monitor) for exercise
- Last cardiologist/internist check-up 2 months ago, no diagnostic findings
- Previous blood tests show no abnormalities (normal hormone status)
- Health-conscious diet according to government guidelines)
- Fluid intake: approximately 0.5 l coffee per day as well as 2.5 l mineral water, up to 3.5 l when exercising, rarely consumes alcohol
- Climacteric problems (hot flashes, increasing mood fluctuations)
- Increasing exhaustion
- Lack of mental alertness
- Increasing fatigue, lack of motivation
- Sleeps well

Personal commentary:

In the last few months I have been feeling increasingly overwhelmed by everyday challenges. My exercise program has not changed. I regularly run 4-5x per week for 45-60 min at a moderate pace. There have been no changes in my personal life. My daughters are in college, so I am able to focus completely on my job, which has always been fun and fulfilling. As a woman, I am very grateful and feel privileged to be on the board and to be in charge of so many associates. But lately I have been at my limit mentally and physically. I am physically fit but not very resilient. I have heard very good things about "Prescription for Energy" from some of my business partners. Something seems to not be working optimally in my body. My last hormone status at the internist's office was normal. A comprehensive analysis of possible deficient substances done by another specialist was inconclusive. The anti-aging specialist thought he could improve my current condition with a targeted hormone intake. I strictly reject that type of treatment. There are no long-term studies. Since I have seen my business partner's results, I have been on fire. I tell myself that this will be the concept to help me. Compared to my colleagues, my diet is quite good. I will start by doing simple saliva tests 4x per day to establish a diurnal stress profile (cortisol).

First test results

My results are evaluated with respect to my age, height, physical activity, and described health problems.

- The cortisol stress hormone profile shows a very stressed vegetative nervous system.
- My three-day acid-base profile shows a primarily alkaline metabolic state and thus offers good micronutrient absorption ability.
- My thyroid hormone levels are borderline, with a tendency to hypofunction. I am astounded because my last medial check-up six months ago supposedly did not require any action.
- My functional energy metabolism shows some abnormalities, high concentration of an acid I am unable to pronounce properly [alpha-ketoglutaric acid] which, as was explained to me, can lead to premature mental fatigue.
- Of note also are some low amino acid concentrations that are very important to the endocrine system.
- My ferritin concentration is very low for physically active women even though I did not menstruate prior to the test date.
- There is a definite optimization requirement for some micronutrients that are measured intracellular rather than in the serum or whole blood.

I mention this specifically because the results from my preliminary tests showed no deficiencies.

The comprehensive analyses make the preparation of an individualized formula possible. It looks as follows:

Prescription for Energy for a 48-year-old woman (BOD HR)

Active ingredient	Daily dose	Active ingredient	Daily dose
Vitamins		**Trace elements**	
Vitamin A (retinol)	1 mg	Chromium	100 µq
Vitamin B_1 (thiamine)	20 mg	Manganese	10 mg
Vitamin B_2 (riboflavin)	20 mg	Copper	4 mg
Vitamin B_6 (pyridoxine)	40 mg	Selenium	150 µq
Vitamin B_{12} (cyanocobalamine)	380 µq	Zinc	48 mg
Vitamin C (ascorbic acid)	1,500 µq	**Minerals**	
Vitamin D_3	30 µq	Calcium	200 mg
Natural vitamin E	200 g	Potassium	100 mg
Of that alpha tocopherol	174.1 mg	Silicon	20 mg
		Quasi-vitamins	
Gama tocopherol	20 mg	Choline	160 mg
Natural carotenoids	8 mg	Coenzyme Q_{10}	90 mg
Of that alpha carotene	80 µq	Inositol	120 mg
		L-carnitine	200 mg
Beta carotene	1.9 mg	PABA	40 mg
Cryptoxanthin	15 µq	**Plant extracts**	
Lutein	8.0 mg	Green tea extract	350.8 mg
Zeaxanthin	15.0 g	Citrus bioflavonoid	200.5 mg
Biotin (vitamin H)	100 mg	Red wine extract	350.8 mg
Folic acid (vitamin B_9)	1.6 mg	**Dietary fiber**	
Niacin (vitamin B_3)	20 mg	Guar gum	3,117.8 mg
Pantothenic acid	40 mg	HPM cellulose	139.6 mg

Additional amino acids in special cases
Arginine 2,000 mg

HCK prescription No: 12689210
Intraday volume 29 ml
(2.9 measuring scoops)

Intake:
½ of daily dose in the morning 1.45
½ of daily does in the afternoon 1.45

Additionally:
- Morning: Iodine 10 min before breakfast
- Afternoon: amino acids as per prescription (activates hormone and brain metabolism).
- Iron supplements at night with dinner 4 x per week (Mon, Wed, Fri, Sun).
- 300 mg magnesium micropellets, let dissolve on tongue.

Fig. 96

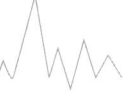

Personal commentary after four months of Prescription for Energy

After four months of Prescription for Energy, I feel like a new person. I am no longer tired and feel like a million dollars. I am better able to handle stress. This is also reflected in the clearly positive progressions of the measured stress hormones (see fig. 97). My mental fitness has improved to the point that my severe overload symptoms from just a few months ago have disappeared. My menopausal symptoms are barely noticeable. This really surprises me. I did not think that so many positive changes could occur in such a short period of time. For me personally this concept for success is ingenius, and I can recommend to other executives to start using it early so they won't even get into a situation like the one I experienced.

Experience after using "Prescription for Energy" for a total of four years

After using this concept for four years, not only do my colleagues on the board of directors benefit from this energy concept, but also second and third level executives in our company, and they are thrilled. We regularly have our energy status measured 1x a year and our formulas adjusted according to the current facts and conditions. Over the past four years, our company has experienced a fabulous trend. I would have never expected my colleagues to turn so euphoric. Mental performance capacity has increased enormously, and we are using our newfound energy for innovative projects. Many more executives in other companies will benefit from these extraordinary positive experiences in the future. I am convinced that with this method overload reactions in executives will be prevented from the start.

Here are my test results

I was diagnosed with a latent hypothyroidism. I now take 1 x Jodid 100 in the morning, 10 minutes before breakfast until the next check-up. Of the HCK blend that was prepared for me by a pharmacist, I take 1.4 measuring scoops in the morning with breakfast. My ferritin level is definitely low and in spite of exercise can lead to increasing fatigue. This was true in my case. For this reason I have to take an iron supplement at night with dinner. One hour before I go to bed I let 300 mg of micropellet magnesium dissolve on my tongue. In this way optimal absorption already occurs in part through the oral muscosa.

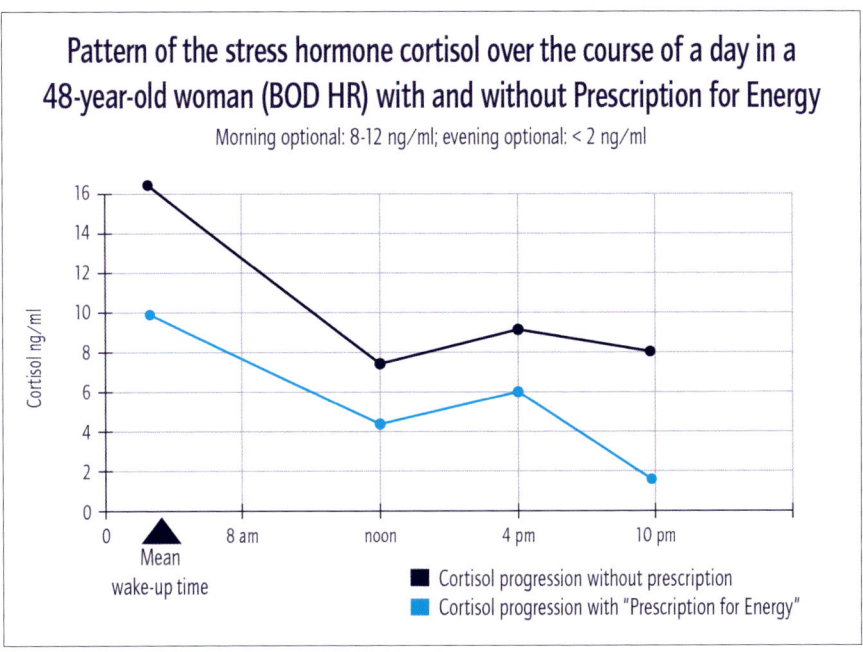

Fig. 97

I was astonished that it is possible to measure the functional energy metabolism with this concept. My levels show one considerably elevated acid (alpha-ketoglutaric acid) and an elevated pyruvate concentration. It was explained to me that initially six different acids and metabolic products would be measured that can show which impairments or biochemical disorders are present in my body. Fig. 98 shows that the dark blue bars touch the red ones, and these are the two referenced values. After four months of Prescription for Energy the light blue bars show that all areas have normalized (see fig. 98). I can now see how the entire micronutrient spectrum is above 20% of mean values (see fig. 99), namely with data based on people of my age, lifestyle, and disorders. This is of critical importance for the evaluation of my results.

The laboratories take measurements, but those can only be evaluated accurately if my personal circumstances are taken into account. Due to the individualized Prescription for Energy formula, definite changes are now apparent (see fig. 99, 100, 101). For me personally, as a rational human being, the severe reduction of stress hormones (with simple saliva samples in the course of the day) by the use of the individualized formula is the best attestation to the concept's uniqueness and effectiveness (see fig. 98).

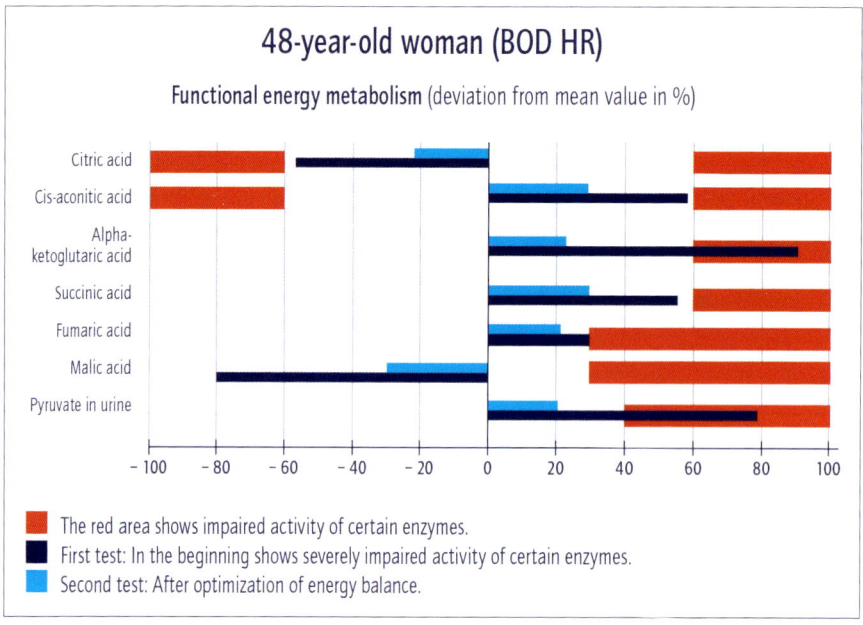

Fig. 98

ANALYSIS AND REGULATION

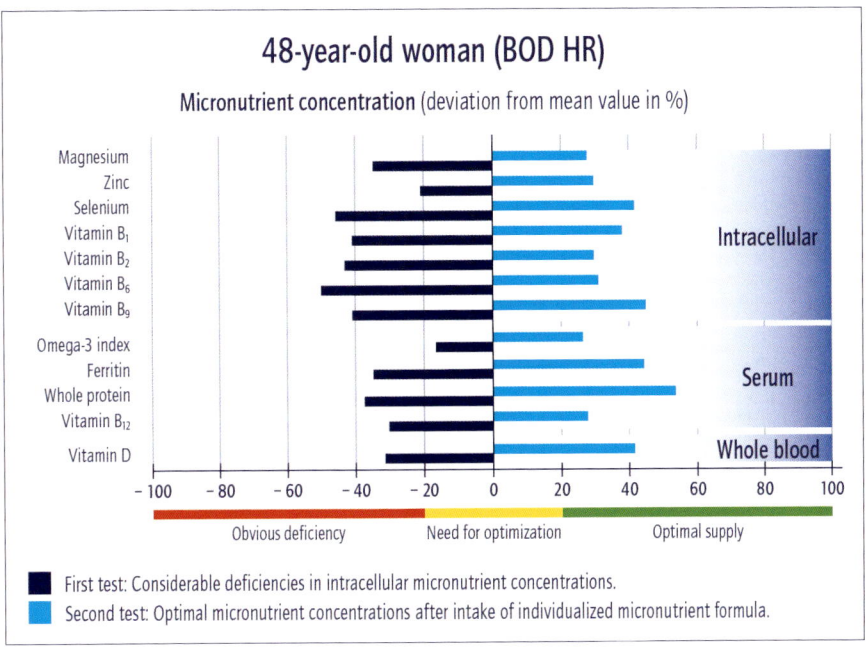

Fig. 99

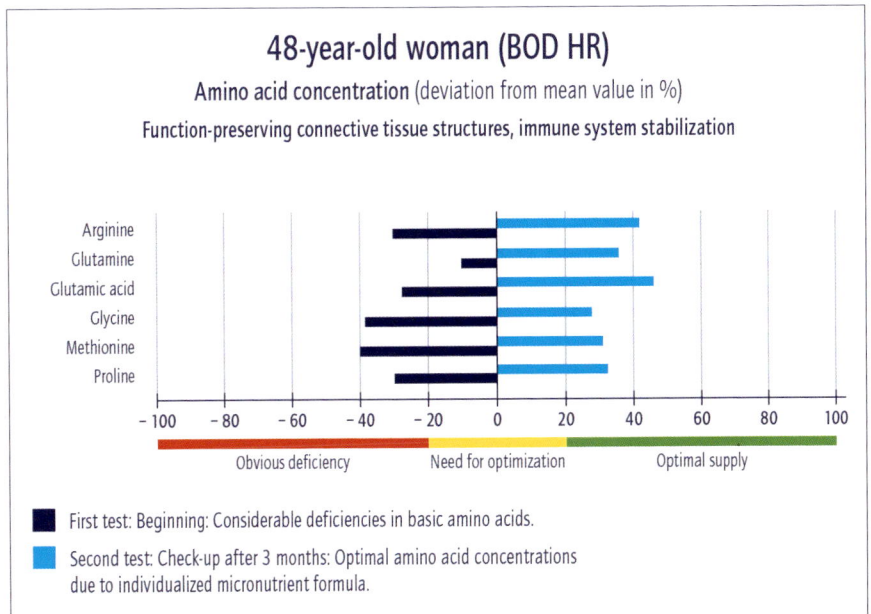

Fig. 100

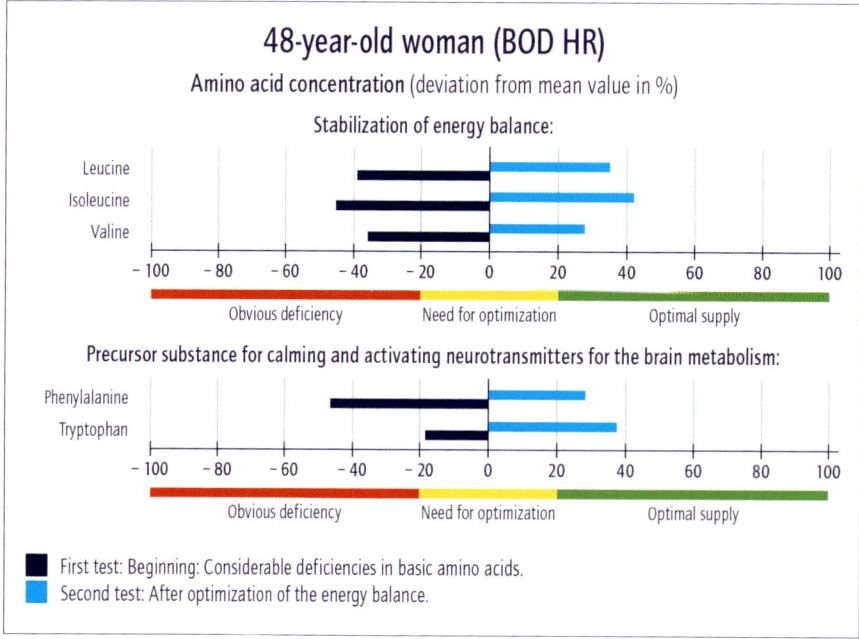

Fig. 101

EXAMPLE CASE OF A 45-YEAR-OLD EXECUTIVE

The completed anamnesis resulted in the following clinical presentation:

- Industrial engineer, general manager – Finance, of a metalworking company with 8,500 associates, married, 2 children
- Height: 6'3"
- Weight: 209.4 lbs
- Former competitive athlete: handball (until age 29); exercising again for last 3 years)
- Jogs for 45 min. 3x per week (with heart rate monitor)
- Last cardiologist/internist check-up 6 months ago: no diagnostic findings
- Previous blood tests show no abnormalities
- Normally health-conscious diet; on business trips doesn't always have the time to watch his diet
- Fluid intake: approximately 0.5 l of coffee per day as well as mineral water, up to 2.5 l when exercising, rarely consumes alcohol
- Increasing exhaustion
- Increased agitation, considerably higher irritability
- Considerably lower stress tolerance
- Trouble sleeping

Personal commentary

I love my job, the level of responsibility, the communication with co-workers, working as a team, and the permanent professional challenges abroad. For the last three years I have been jogging regularly 2-3x per week for approximately 45 minutes, without getting competitive with myself. I am happily married; have two children (ages: 3 and 5). Lately I have noticed a lack of mental fitness (poor concentration ability during the day), I have light night sweats, am often tired in the evening, feel somewhat agitated during the day, and lose my inner composure—of course I don't let it show on the outside. I go to sleep easily at night but don't sleep through the night. I keep waking up. I also feel increased mood fluctuations. Progressive muscle relaxation or autogenic training, which were recommended and arranged by a therapist, did not result in any change. After jogging I sometimes get a calf cramp. I therefore take magnesium regularly. My wife recently told me that I seem very stressed and no longer seem as even-tempered as I used to be. She got me some vitamins at the pharmacy, which I would take in the morning. They were not cheap, but the ailments did not really improve. On the contrary, I slept even worse than before. I don't know why this was the case. A physician friend told me: "You can throw these in the trash. They won't do anything and just cost money!"

First test results

The results were evaluated with respect to my age, height, sex, prior illnesses, physical activity, and the described health problems.

- My thyroid hormones show a tendency to hypofunction. But from a medical standpoint there is no action required.
- The expensive vitamin supplements I got from my wife are counterproductive because they contain additional iodine and increase my agitation.
- My functional energy metabolism shows impaired activity of certain enzymes that has lead to biochemical disorders.
- An amino acid whose name I have trouble recalling [tryptophan] is definitely deficient. This is significant with respect to my sleep issues and increasing mood fluctuations.
- My omega-3 index is very low and thus can worsen increasing mood fluctuations.
- Good mental fitness is only possible at 20% above the mean values of individual micronutrients. I am considerably lower than that compared to comparable people of my age (even though my previous test done by my family physician did not show any abnormalities).

Personal commentary after three months of Prescription for Energy

After completing three months of Prescription for Energy I feel transformed. At the beginning I experienced some slight flatulence. But that stopped after two weeks. My wife told me: "You are much more even-tempered even though your job-related stress has increased." She is right, as I handle occurring stressors much more calmly and now even keep my composure during absolute stress phases. I am amazed that the nightly dose of the individual amino acid tryptophan, whose name will always sound exotic to my ears, has such a positive effect on my sleep behavior. After approximately five days I was able to sleep much better, and that without medication. The individualized micronutrient formula definitely decreased the alpha-ketoglutaric acid level. This sounds as though I have become an expert, but by now you can see that I have understood some relationships. An increase in this acid means increased central fatigue.

Experience after using Prescription for Energy for a total of five years

I am absolutely thrilled by the Prescription for Energy concept. For five years now I have my energy status checked 1x per year, and depending on my current status, I receive an adjusted formula. This in particular is fantastic, that the prescription is adjusted to my personal circumstances. In the meantime many of my business partners have benefitted from this unique concept. Since then increasing exhaustion or lacking mental fitness is a thing of the past. My desire: to preserve my health and performance capacity by early detection of biochemical disorders and their correction. In our extremely demanding job this is the way of the future! A true pioneering feat, and with fantastic results for me!

7.3 CASE STUDIES OF TOP COMPETITIVE ATHLETES

EXAMPLE CASE OF A 34-YEAR-OLD SELF-EMPLOYED MALE

The completed anamnesis resulted in the following clinical presentation:

- Self-employed, retirement planning service provider, three coworkers, married, 2 children
- Height: 5'8"
- Weight: 147.7 lbs
- Competitive athlete: physically very active, burnout with hospitalization and antidepressants after running a marathon
- Last cardiologist/internist check-up three weeks ago
- Previous blood tests show no abnormalities
- Health-conscious diet according to government guidelines
- Fluid intake: approximately 0.5 l coffee per day, as well as 3.5 l mineral water, up to 4 l with physical activity, no alcohol
- Very stressful job; many good new clients with increasing revenue
- Agitation
- Isolated anxiety-attacks in spite of medication
- Lack of mental alertness
- Poor sleep quality

Personal commentary

Since I became self-employed two years ago, I have been able to attract many new clients, which has given me a sound financial base. Ten to thirteen hour workdays are the norm and are fun even though my job-related stress was already near the limit. Since I have always been ambitious I decided to run the Berlin marathon in under 2 ½ hours. Since I used to get very good running times on shorter distances in the past, this goal was realistic. Every minute of my day was planned out. My wife and children supported my undertaking. I had to carve out 15-20 hours per week for training to reach my goal. Then the day came, and I was actually able to reach this goal, but with the consequence of a subsequent hospitalization after several panic attacks at night. I was no longer able to relax without psychotropic drugs and no longer had any quality of life. My batteries are still completely dead. Then I read an article by Dr. Wienecke in a Tv-magazine on the topic job—sports—burnout, and I immediately thought: This energy concept will help me get back to my old life.

First test results

The "batteries" in my body are completely dead; certain measurements show major demands on the body's own structural proteins.

- I have a tendency to hypothyroidism. A TSH-base value of < 1.3 µIU/ml can verifiably lead to severe stress of the vegetative nervous system (sympathicotonia). This considerably reduces the replenishment of certain glycogen stores in the liver and musculature and rapidly leads to overload reactions.
- My functional energy metabolism shows significantly impaired activity of certain enzymes, which has resulted in the inhibition of the entire system.
- A certain acid that is considerably elevated has caused significant ammoniac accumulation, triggering increasing central fatigue.
- Of particular note are the low concentrations of some amino acids that are important to brain metabolism.
- Also of note are the considerably low intracellular magnesium and B vitamin concentrations.

Personal commentary after six weeks of Prescription for Energy

After six weeks of Prescription for Energy I have phenomenal news. Even if my wife says that I am currently a walking biogas plant, the progression is almost unbelievable. I modified my diet according to the recommendations and surprisingly no longer had any craving for sweets, which I used to consume large amounts of.

My health also continues to improve. After only three weeks, I was able to lower my antidepressant dosage (against panic attacks) by half and after six weeks discontinued it completely. The severe panic attacks are now completely gone. I would have never thought such a quick reaction possible. In summary I would say that I haven't felt this good in a year.

To the director and associates of SALUTO: You should broaden your finding and experience to the sphere of mental health. A professor at the university hospital in Münster, Germany, whom I told about your theories within the context of a treatment, dismissed these with the words: "Nutrition has nothing to do with the psyche; this is not substantiated!" We'll see what he has to say when I tell him next month that I'm doing just fine without psychotropic drugs.

After my personal walk through hell I am very grateful and glad to have learned about the ingenius Prescription for Energy concept by chance. I am convinced that this method is the way of the future. Don't wait until things get so bad that you end up in a situation like mine!

EXAMPLE CASE OF A 22-YEAR-OLD PRO-SOCCER PLAYER FROM A TOP ITALIAN TEAM

The completed anamnesis resulted in the following clinical presentation:

- Previous cardiologist/internist check-up 2 months ago: no diagnostic findings
- Previous blood tests show no abnormalities
- Health-conscious diet according to government guidelines
- Fluid intake: approximately 0.5 l coffee per day, as well as 3.5 l mineral water with a high hydrogen carbonate concentration (> 1,500 mg/l)
- Increased illnesses that have resulted in training interruptions
- Increasing exhaustion with performance fluctuations
- Lack of mental alertness
- Frequent fatigue

Personal commentary

My trainer told me that my performance potential has not been fully tapped and that I have the prospect of playing a central role on the national team. I completed all of the stages of youth and junior national teams with flying colors. But in the last 1 ½ years repeated illnesses have resulted in missed training. For the past six months I have felt a lack of mental alertness and am experiencing increasing exhaustion that has lead to performance fluctuations. I have heard from many of my teammates who have been using Prescription for Energy for longer periods of time, and have been able to achieve exceptional success in their performance development. Italy does perform detailed analyses, but mine did not show any abnormalities. But I am certain that with this currently unique testing method my performance development and mental alertness can be optimized, and that my aspiration to start on the national team will then be achievable.

Prescription for Energy for a 22-year-old pro soccer player (national team player)

Active ingredient	Daily dose	Active ingredient	Daily dose
Vitamins		Trace elements	
Vitamin A (retinol)	1 mg	Chromium	250 µq
Vitamin B_1 (thiamine)	50 mg	Manganese	10 mg
Vitamin B_2 (riboflavin)	30 mg	Copper	4 mg
Vitamin B_6 (pyridoxine)	40 mg	Selenium	200 µq
Vitamin B_{12} (cyanocobalamine)	780 µq	Zinc	48 mg
Vitamin C (ascorbic acid)	1,500 µq	**Minerals**	
Vitamin D_3	55 µq	Calcium	200 mg
Natural vitamin E	200 g	Potassium	400 mg
Of that alpha tocopherol	174.1 mg	Magnesium	300 mg
		Silicon	40 mg
Gama tocopherol	20 mg	**Quasi-vitamins**	
Natural carotenoids	8 mg	Choline	200 mg
Of that alpha carotene	80 µq	Coenzyme Q_{10}	120 mg
		Inositol	120 mg
Beta carotene	1.9 mg	L-carnitine	500 mg
Cryptoxanthin	15 µq	PABA	40 mg
Lutein	6.0 mg	**Plant extracts**	
Zeaxanthin	15.0 g	Green tea extract	350.8 mg
Biotin (vitamin H)	100 mg	Citrus bioflavonoid	260.5 mg
Folic acid (vitamin B_9)	2 mg	Red wine extract	380.8 mg
Niacin (vitamin B_3)	40 mg	**Dietary fiber**	
Pantothenic acid	60 mg	Guar gum	3,517.8 mg
		HPM cellulose	145.6 mg

Additional amino acids in special cases	
Arginine	3,000 mg

HCK prescription No: 12688920
Intraday volume 35 ml
(3.4 measuring scoops)

Intake:
Morning ½ of daily dosage 1.7
Afternoon ½ of daily dosage 1.7

Additionally:
- Morning: Iodine 10 min before breakfast
- Morning and Afternoon: Omega-3 fatty acids 2 capsules morning and afternoon (a capsule contains: 300 mg EPA and 200 DHA).
- 60 g of a complex amino acid blend with a high percentage of collagen peptides (arginine, methionine, proline)
- Intake 20 g before 1st training, 20 g directly after 1st training and 20 g after the 2nd training.
- 300 mg magnesium in micropellet form dissolved on the tongue.

Fig. 102

My first test results

- The "batteries" in my body are completely dead; certain measurements show major demands on the body's own structural proteins (pyridinium crosslinks) and severe depletion.
- I have a tendency to hypothyroidism. A TSH-basal value of 3.3 µIU/ml can verifiably lead to increasing central fatigue. In competitive athletes a TSH-basal value of > 2.8 already results in worse regeneration after intense exertion (feeling of increasing fatigue).
- My functional energy metabolism shows severe activity impairment in certain enzymes that has resulted in inhibition of the entire system.
- One of the acids is considerably elevated (alpha-ketoglutaric acid). I was told that this has resulted in major ammoniac accumulation, causing increasing fatigue.
- Of particular note are the low concentrations of some amino acids that are important to brain metabolism. Of note are the considerably low arginine and tryptophan concentrations. The latter can also explain my fluctuating moods.

Personal comments after four months of Prescription for Energy

After taking Prescription for Energy for four months I feel transformed. I possess a mental alertness I haven't felt for a long time in recent years. To me personally this concept for success is genius, and I can recommend to other players to start using this early so they don't even experience a situation like mine. My performance in the club is better than ever. I notice that I regenerate much better after intense training and competitive exertions. After the first four months the initial criticism from my support staff, particularly our team physician, has all but vanished as I now continuously show exceptional performances in the club.

Experience after using "Prescription for Energy" for a total of two years

After a two-year use I am able to tap my full performance potential. I have my energy status checked 2x per year and receive a newly adjusted formula. The leap into the A-national team worked out. No training loss due to illness and other minor overload reactions like the ones I used to experience in the past. Meanwhile all of my teammates in the club benefit from this unique concept for success, and I can say without exaggeration that it is essential for every elite athlete. Every athlete has an individual energy requirement. With the special analyses any complex biochemical disorders will be detected and corrected early. Even my support team is now totally enthusiastic. Italy, in particular, has always valued medical assistance.

Here is a brief summary of some of my results

I was diagnosed with latent hypothyroidism. I now take 2x Jodid 100 in the morning, 10 minutes before breakfast until the next check-up.

Of the HCK-blend that a pharmacist prepared for me I take 1.6 measuring scoops in the morning and 1.6 measuring scoops in the afternoon with food. Initially my gastrointestinal tract had to get used to this intake as I had increased flatulence. After two weeks it was gone. I was astonished that my amino acids deviated so much from the mean values of comparable players with my disorders. For this reason I take 20 g before the first training, directly after the first training, and after the second training each day. What is important for me here is not the total protein, but the quality of collagen peptides (special proteins that stabilize connective tissue). My levels show a significantly elevated acid (alpha-ketoglutaric acid), which explained my initial fatigue during intense training and competition phases. Fig. 103 shows that the dark blue bar reaches the red area and that after four months this acid verifiably normalized (light blue bar). In the beginning my body had to use its own substance so I could tolerate training and competition-related stress. After four months of Prescription for Energy this stress has verifiably diminished (see fig. 104). In the long-term the optimization of my energy balance (especially the replenishing of intracellular micronutrient concentrations) leads to a significantly decreased demand on the body's own structural proteins. This all sounds very appealing, but it shows my progression. And that is how I am feeling.

ANALYSIS AND REGULATION

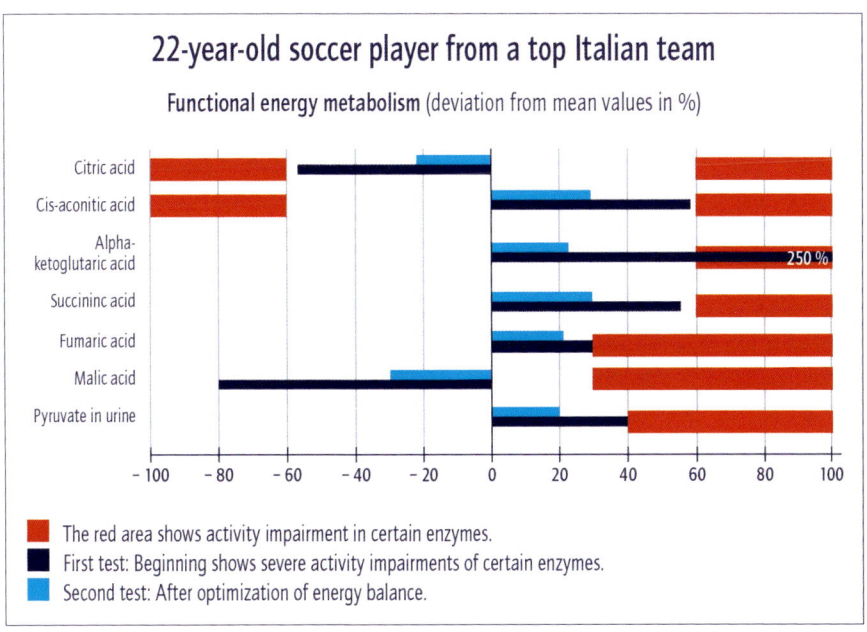

Fig. 103

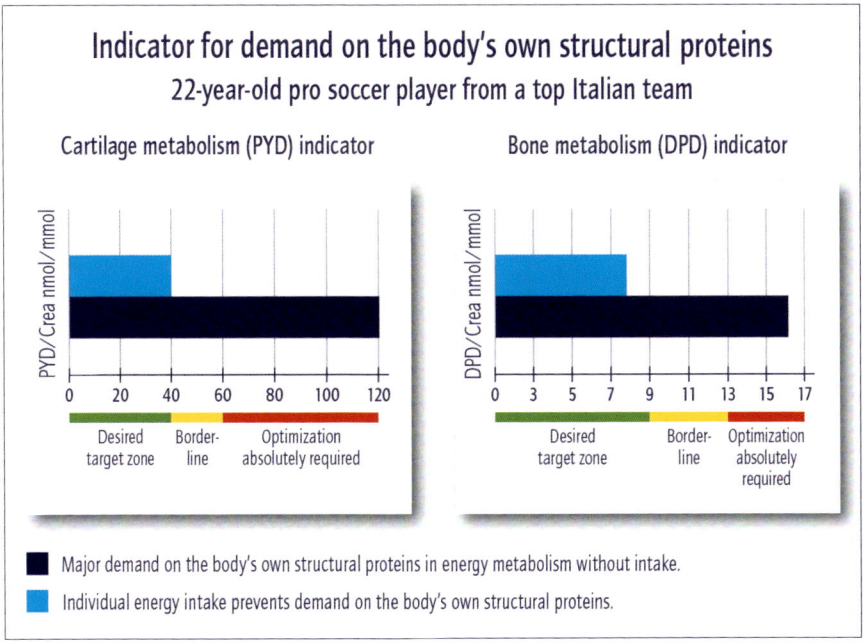

Fig. 104

EXAMPLE CASE OF THE GERMAN HANDBALL FEDERATION'S YOUTH AND JUNIOR NATIONAL TEAM OF 72 PLAYERS TOTAL OVER A PERIOD OF SIX YEARS (EUROPEAN YOUTH CHAMPIONS 2008, JUNIOR NATIONAL CHAMPIONS 2009 AND 2011, EUROPEAN YOUTH CHAMPIONS 2012)

The players received a comprehensive check-up 2x per year, within the scope of a one-of-a-kind European concept for prevention by SALUTO with the DHB (German Handball Federation) and the HDZ (Heart and Diabetes Center NRW Bad Oeynhausen, Germany). Along with neuromuscular coordination tests, biomechanical function analyses, flexibility tests, various strength tests, sprint and jump tests, reaction and speed index, field-based step tests, cardiology and internal medicine tests, and dental exams, a comprehensive analysis of the respective energy potential of each individual player was completed.

The first step: Functional energy metabolism analysis, intracellular micronutrient analysis, amino acids and pyridinium crosslinks (indicator for the use of the body's own structural proteins), comparison with the data bank, and the timing of the training and competition phase.

At the beginning of the pilot project, the players reported:
- Lack of mental and physical alertness
- Frequent performance fluctuations during the season
- Increasing fatigue
- Problems concentrating
- Poor regeneration after intense training and competition-related exertion
- Frequent training loss due to increasing illnesses

Each player received a customized formula (Prescription for Energy) that was derived from the comprehensive analyses (see fig. 105). The functional energy metabolism analysis and the pyridinium crosslinks (see fig. 105) were measured 4x per year. After the analysis each player received a modified and adjusted formula. After Prescription for Energy, the pyridinium crosslinks results no longer show long-term demand on the body's own structural proteins that lead to premature depletion, as was frequently the case at the beginning of the pilot project.

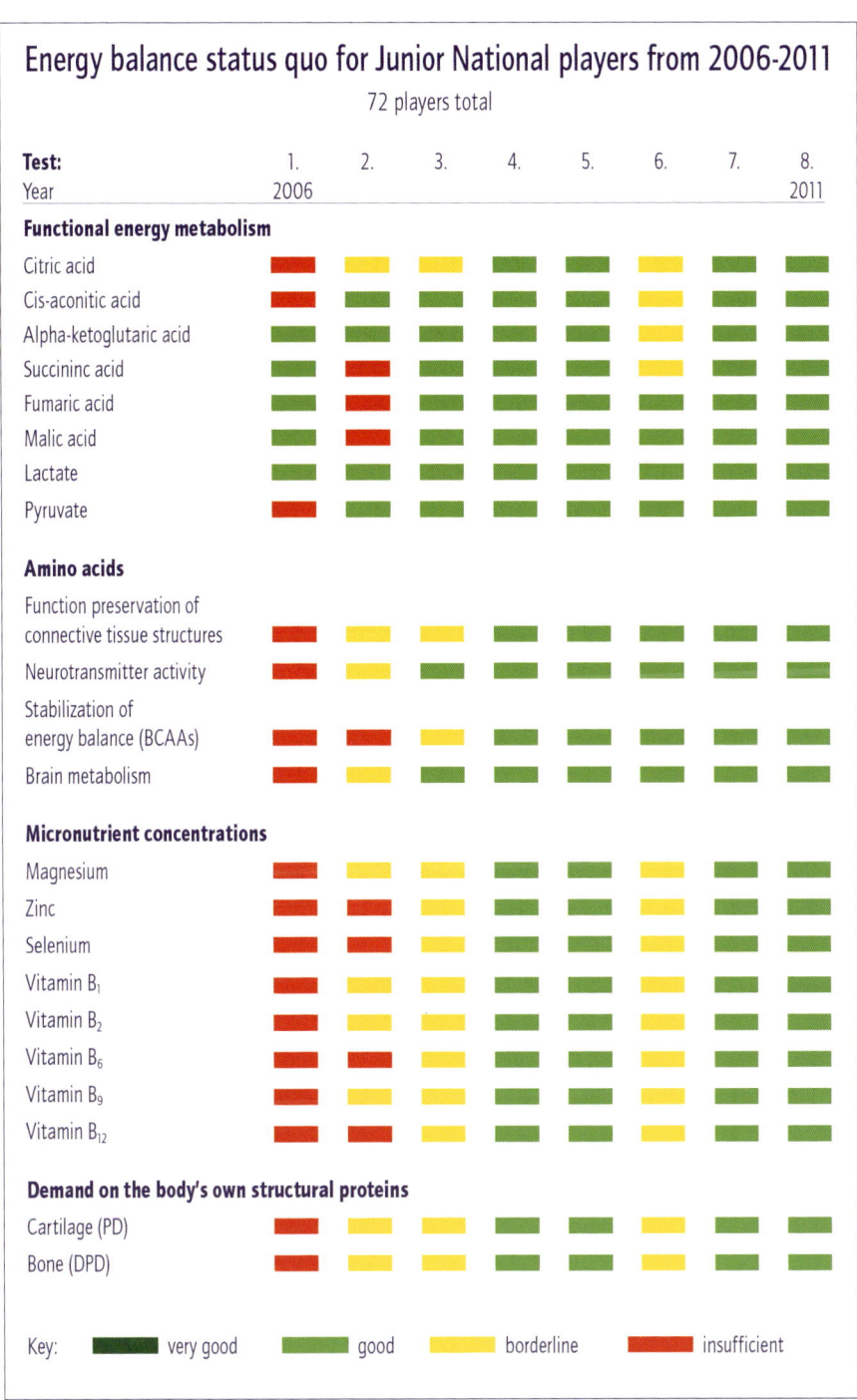

Fig. 105

Because of Prescription for Energy the various disorders the players reported in the beginning could no longer be detected over the course of the project. On the contrary, the players showed significant improvement in their mental and physical fitness (exception: Army basic training during 6th test).

Here is a summary of some comments:
- Player A: Faster regeneration, easier to wake up, better concentration.
- Player B: Good regeneration, considerably improved mental fitness also during training courses, no more illnesses like in the past.
- Player C: "Many of my teammates and myself are absolutely convinced that we became 2011 Junior World champions because we were able to regenerate from the games so unbelievably fast. Since I started taking the micronutrients I feel transformed and super-resilient!"
- Player D: Steadily improved tolerance; no more problems after a month of "Prescription for Energy". Since then few if any injuries; feeling of increasing body stability and strength; at first haltingly, then increasingly definite refreshing and vitalizing effect.
- Player E: Faster regeneration, hardly any muscle soreness, good recovery, fewer illnesses, less fatigue, slightly unsettled stomach.
- Player F: "Better physical feeling; I feel alert, fresher, and more focused. Since I started taking micronutrients my susceptibility to injury has verifiably decreased."
- Player G: "Before the European Youth championships last summer I had concerns regarding the stress since I had never played in a tournament like that. With the micronutrient intake I was able to regenerate after all the games and was simply in better shape. The European championship title ultimately confirms that we stayed one step ahead of our opponents. I am about to graduate from high school and with that workload in addition to handball, being stressed is inevitable. With the micronutrient intake I was able to considerably improve my ability to concentrate."

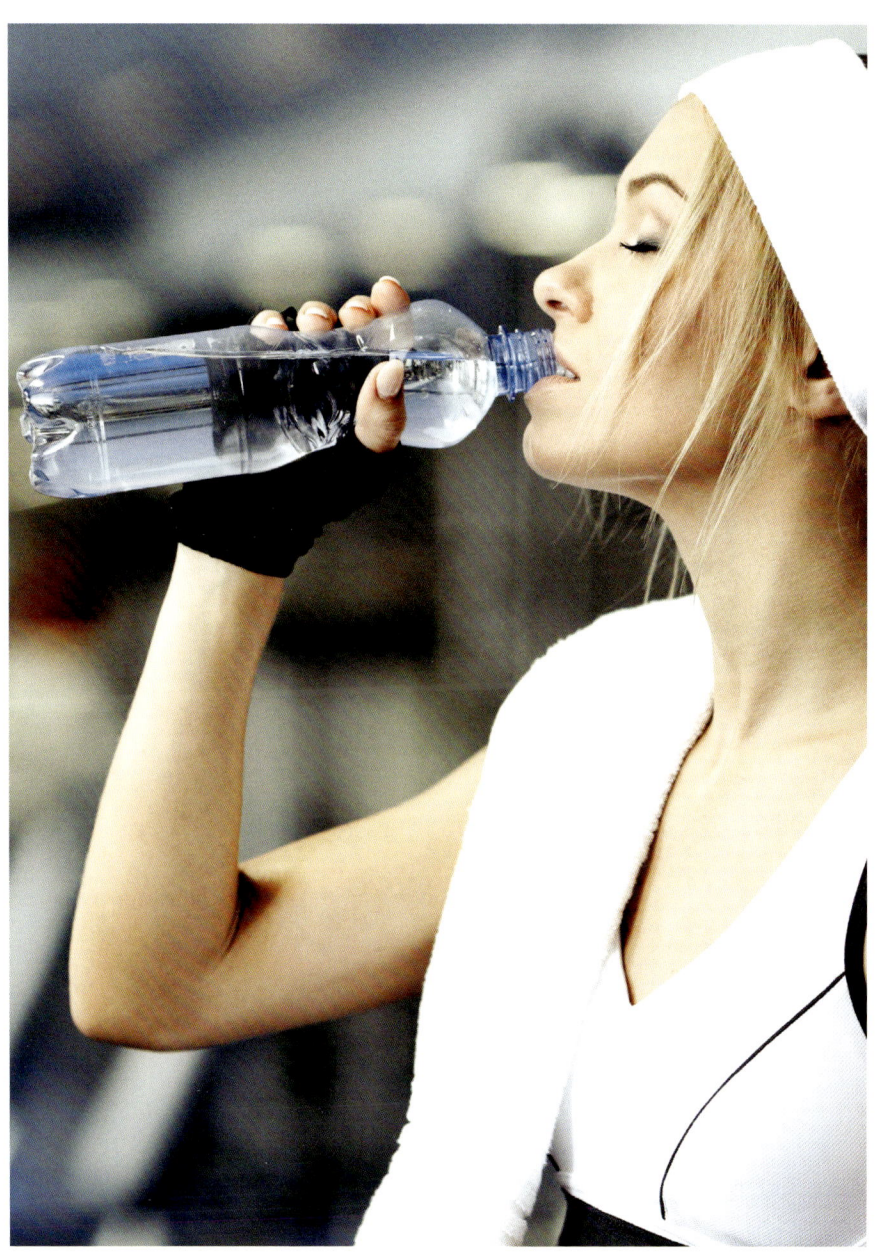

7.4 COMMENTS ON PRESCRIPTION FOR ENERGY

ENTREPRENEUR: AGE 53; 4,600 ASSOCIATES

"My top-tier and second-tier executives as well as myself have benefitted from this unique concept for four years. We are absolutely thrilled and have our energy status checked regularly at least 1x per year, with the goal of having each individual's formula adjusted to his current requirement."

GENERAL MANAGER: AGE 45; 2,800 ASSOCIATES

"I feel good, healthy, and highly productive since I have gotten my individualized micronutrient formula. No more mood fluctuations or that burned out feeling. Three months after the targeted intake I also don't have any more problems with hay fever (primarily grasses)—no watery eyes, no swollen nasal tissue. It's a whole new quality of life."

ENTREPRENEUR: AGE 57; 11,900 ASSOCIATES

"Increasing exhaustion, major mood fluctuations, the feeling of being overwhelmed as an entrepreneur—all of these side-effects have disappeared. I have been using Prescription for Energy for three years. It is a unique concept for success that has restored my quality of life. I am certain that in the near future many companies, but also private individuals, will benefit from this ingenius concept."

NATIONAL TEAM SOCCER PLAYER FROM ITALY

"I am finally able to tap my full potential. I regenerate much quicker and feel mentally great in the Champions League in spite of the demands. My trainer approached me and asked about the comprehensive analyses and my complete formula. I would not have thought that Prescription for Energy could have such a positive effect on my performance capacity. In the meantime some teammates on the national team are also benefitting from this concept."

ENTREPRENEUR: AGE 49

"Since I began using this concept I feel absolutely balanced, am able to sleep exceptionally well, and feel like a different person. Companies, but also the insurance companies, should embrace this "energy concept" in order to achieve enormous savings potential in the future."

DHB (GERMAN HANDBALL FEDERATION) JUNIOR WORLD CHAMPION

"I have been using Prescription for Energy and have been able to celebrate astonishing success. In the past I have had frequent mood fluctuations and repeated minor injuries during intense training and competition phases. I have had my energy status measured 4x per year, and my formula was adjusted each time. I am convinced that the future of elite sports will include the use of this concept so that near-limit athletic exertion can be tolerated better. Meantime many of my fellow players are absolutely thrilled."

ANDREAS TÖLZER: VICE-WORLD CHAMPION; EUROPEAN CHAMPION; MULTIPLE GERMAN CHAMPION (MARTIAL ARTS)

"In recent years I had repeated illnesses and minor injuries prior to important competitions—the Olympic games, world and European championships—that prevented me from tapping my full performance potential. Since I began using Prescription for Energy, I have not been sick or had injuries and have been extraordinarily successful. Many more athletic successes would have been possible if I had used this concept for success years ago."

APPENDIX

1 BIBLIOGRAPHICAL REFERENCES

This book addresses many themes, but to discuss them scientifically would go beyond the scope of this book. For additional information, please refer to the following bibliographical reference list. Our intent for this book is to raise awareness in executives (entrepreneurs, executive managers, executive staff), and top competitive athletes regarding the Prescription for Energy concept.

- Addis, P., Shecterle, L. M. & Alexander, J. (2012). Cellular protection during oxidative stress: A potential role for d-ribose and antioxidants. *J Diet Suppl, 9 (3)*. 178-82.

- Dickhuth, H. H., Mayer, F., Röcker K. & Berg A. (Hrsg.). (2007). *Sportmedizin für Ärzte – Lehrbuch auf der Grundlage des Weiterbildungssystems der Deutschen Gesellschaft für Sportmedizin und Prävention (DGSP).* Deutscher Ärzte Verlag. Köln.

- Feil, W. & Wessinghage, T. (2008). *Ernährung und Training – 20 Bausteine für Ihre Fitness.* (7. Aufl.). WESSP. Nürnberg.

- Fischer, G., Eichenberg, C., Mosetter, K. & Mosetter, R. (2006). *Stress im Beruf.* Asanger. Heidelberg.

- Geue, B. (2006). *Autogenes Training und Muskelentspannung.* 2 Kassetten in Duo Box. Trias. Stuttgart.

- Graf, C. & Höher, J. (2008). *Fachlexikon Sportmedizin für Ärzte – Bewegung Fitness Ernährung von A-Z.* Deutscher Ärzteverlag. Köln.

- Hamm, M. (2007). *Brainfood: Fitmacher für kluge Köpfe.* (2. Aufl.). Mosaik. Berlin.

- Mosetter, K. & Mosetter, R. (2003). *Kraft in der Dehnung. Ein Praxisbuch bei Stress, Dauerbelastung und Trauma.* (5. Aufl. 2007). Patmos. Düsseldorf, Zürich.

- Dies. (2008). *Schmerzen heilen mit der KiD-Methode. Der achtsame Umgang mit dem eigenen Körper.* Patmos. Düsseldorf.

- Dies. (2008). Traumatische Belastungen: Der Körper als Bühne und szenische Macht. *ZPPM, 1.* 8-24.

- Dies. (2010). *Myoreflextherapie Band 2. Regulation für Körper, Gehirn und Erleben.* Vesalius. Konstanz.

- Mosetter, K. (2008). Chronischer Stress auf der Ebene der Molekularbiologie und Neurobiochemie. In: G. Fischer & P. Schay (Hrsg.). *Psychodynamische Psycho- und Traumatherapie. Konzepte – Praxis – Perspektiven.* VS Verlag für Sozialwissenschaften. Wiesbaden.

- Mosetter, K., Pape, D. & Cavelius, A. (2012 [in preparation]). *Die vier Kräfte der Selbstheilung.* Gräfe/Unzer. München.
- Mosetter, K. & Reutter, W. (2007). Insulin und Insulinresistenz im Gehirn. *Schweiz Zschr GaMed, 3.* 138-141.
- Pilz-Kusch, U. (2012). *Burn-out – Frühsignale erkennen – Kraft gewinnen. Das Praxishandbuch für Trainer, Berater und Betroffene.* Beltz Verlag. Weinheim.
- Reglin, F. (2009). *Bausteine des Lebens – Aminosäuren in der orthomolekularen Medizin.* (3. Aufl.). Reglin-Verlag. Köln.
- Reutter, W. & Mosetter, K. (2006). *Zellulärer Stress und Molekulare Antwort.* Vortrag an der Tertianum-Fachtagung: Prävention, Frühintervention und Strategien für ein erfolgreiches Altern. Zürich, 19. Oktober 2006. (www.tertianumzfp.ch). Zürich.
- Roser, M., Josic, D., Kontou, M., Mosetter, K., Maurer, P. & Reutter, W. (2009). Metabolism of galactose in the brain and liver of rats and its conversion into glutamate and other amino acids. *J Neural Transm, 116 (2).* 131-9.
- Ross, J. (2010 Deusche Ausgabe) Was die Seele essen will. *Mood Cure.* S. 359-372, Klatt-Cotta Verlag
- Sapolsky, R. M.; Hrsg. von D. Kahnemann et al. (1999) *In Well Being.* Russel Sage Foundation. New York.
- Schartl, M., Gesseler, M. & von Eckardstein, A. (2009). *Biochemie und Molekularbiologie des Menschen.* (1. Aufl.). Urban & Fischer. München.
- Schmid, S. M., Hallschmid, M., Jauch-Chara, K., Wilms, B., Lehnert, H., Born, J. & Schultes, B. (2011). Disturbed glucoregulatory response to food intake after moderate sleep restriction. *Sleep, 34 (3).* 371-7.
- Schulz, H. & Heck, H. (2006). Laktat und Ammoniakverhalten bei erschöpfenden Dauerbelastungen. 97-107. In: U. Bartmus, G. Jendrusch, T. Heneke & P. Platen (Hrsg.). *In memoriam Horst de Marées anlässlich seines 70. Geburtstags. Beiträge aus Sportmedizin, Trainings- und Bewegungswissenschaft.* Sportverlag Strauß. Köln.
- Teitelbaum, J. E. (2007). *From Fatigued to Fantastic.* New York: Penguin. 31-41, 278.
- Teitelbaum, J. E., Johnson, C. & St Cyr, J. (2006). The use of D-ribose in chronic fatigue syndrome and fibromyalgia: a pilot study. *J Altern Complement Med, 12 (9).* 857-62.
- Wienecke, E. (2011). *Performance Explosion in Sports – An Anti-Doping Concept.* Meyer & Meyer. Aachen.
- Wienecke, E. (2003). *Das Programm für Lebensqualität pur. Fitness für Körper und Geist. Aktiv gegen freie Radikale. Vitamine für die Seele.* Südwest-Verlag. München.

2   INFORMATION ON THE INTERNET (AVAILABLE BY DOWNLOAD)

Various documents and materials from this book as well as additional information can also be found or downloaded from the Internet:

Both self-checks can be downloaded in PDF format at:

www. Energie-auf-Rezept.de

www.saluto.de
www.stiftung-mikronaehrstoffe.de

www.hepart.com
www.unisan.de
www.tempur.de

3   ACKNOWLEDGEMENTS

Successful visionary concepts are only possible with good partners. Many thanks to PD Dr. med. Heinrich Körtke, director of the Institute for Applied Telemedicine at the HDZ NRW (Heart and Diabetes Center Bad Oeynhausen), who decisively influenced the advancement of SALUTO. Thank you also to Prof. Dr. med. Reiner Körfer who, as long-time medical director of the HDZ NRW, has supported our development for 17 years.

Special thanks to the Bertelsmann Foundation, in particular Liz Mohn, who made an important contribution with the screening initiative of her co-workers to the now internationally successful "Prescription for Energy" concept.

A heartfelt thank you to Gerhard Weber, Udo Hardieck, and Ralf Weber who gave advice and supported the development of SALUTO with their life's work, the GERRY WEBER WORLD. We look forward to continuing this successful collaboration.

4 ABOUT SALUTO (SOCIETY FOR SPORT AND HEALTH)

SALUTO was established from the area of sports medicine at the University Bielefeld, Germany. Prof. Dr. Elmar Wienecke is co-founder and owner. With its combination of medical services, diagnostics, science, and research, SALUTO has become an internationally recognized center of competence for health and fitness in Germany.

Over the past 20 years, SALUTO, with the cooperation of the Heart and Diabetes Center NRW Bad Oeynhausen and the Oberhofer & Partner dental practice, has developed a comprehensive study design. 10,570 executives, 11,150 top competitive athletes, as well as 6,150 recreational and 8,750 non-athletes, have undergone comprehensive testing.

The Prescription for Energy concept began to emerge in 2006 from clinical studies and many research projects. The goal of this successful energy concept: The timely detection and correction of biochemical disorders to guarantee health and performance capacity. Meanwhile Olympic athletes, world champions, European champions, and German national champions all benefit from this integrated concept. But many executives have also been successfully using this concept for years.

5 SELF CHECKS: WHAT IS THE STATE OF MY ENERGY BALANCE?

Here you can quickly and easily yourself without the comprehensive blood and urine analyses. Of course this is only a rough orientation. It is not possible to create an individualized formula from this data. To do so would require the special analyses. You can also find the download code for these tests on page 218.

ENERGY SELF-CHECK FOR EXECUTIVES
(ENTREPRENEURS, MANAGERS, EXECUTIVE STAFF)

This self-check includes a series of findings regarding your mental and physical state and/or activities over the past seven days and nights.

Please check all that apply and add up the points.

Over the past seven days or nights . . .

. . . I slept badly.

0	1	2	3	4
Never	Rarely	Repeatedly	Regularly	Always

. . . I had night sweats (unrelated to weather) and my clothing was damp when I woke in the morning.

0	1	2	3	4
Never	Rarely	Repeatedly	Regularly	Always

. . . I felt increasingly tired.

0	1	2	3	4
Never	Rarely	Repeatedly	Regularly	Always

. . . I felt drained and unwell.

0	1	2	3	4
Never	Rarely	Repeatedly	Regularly	Always

. . . I felt agitated during the day.

0	1	2	3	4
Never	Rarely	Repeatedly	Regularly	Always

. . . I quickly lost my composure during stressful phases.

0	1	2	3	4
Never	Rarely	Repeatedly	Regularly	Always

. . . I felt annoyed by others.

0	1	2	3	4
Never	Rarely	Repeatedly	Regularly	Always

. . . I harbored feelings of discord.

0	1	2	3	4
Never	Rarely	Repeatedly	Regularly	Always

. . . I did not feel even-tempered.

0	1	2	3	4
Never	Rarely	Repeatedly	Regularly	Always

. . . I felt physically faint.

0	1	2	3	4
Never	Rarely	Repeatedly	Regularly	Always

. . . I had a headache.

0	1	2	3	4
Never	Rarely	Repeatedly	Regularly	Always

. . . I was in a good mood.

0	1	2	3	4
Never	Rarely	Repeatedly	Regularly	Always

. . . I was dissatisfied with myself.

0	1	2	3	4
Never	Rarely	Repeatedly	Regularly	Always

. . . I put off work.

0	1	2	3	4
Never	Rarely	Repeatedly	Regularly	Always

. . . I woke up during the night for no reason.

0	1	2	3	4
Never	Rarely	Repeatedly	Regularly	Always

. . . I was under pressure to perform.

0	1	2	3	4
Never	Rarely	Repeatedly	Regularly	Always

. . . I felt energized.

0	1	2	3	4
Never	Rarely	Repeatedly	Regularly	Always

. . . I felt like I did not get enough breaks.

0	1	2	3	4
Never	Rarely	Repeatedly	Regularly	Always

. . . I was dissatisfied with my diet.

0	1	2	3	4
Never	Rarely	Repeatedly	Regularly	Always

. . . I had alcohol at night so I could sleep better.

0	1	2	3	4
Never	Rarely	Repeatedly	Regularly	Always

. . . I felt like I might explode during phases of stress (agitation).

0	1	2	3	4
Never	Rarely	Repeatedly	Regularly	Always

. . . I was very indignant when criticized.

0	1	2	3	4
Never	Rarely	Repeatedly	Regularly	Always

. . . I ate 600-800 g of fruit and vegetables every day.

0	1	2	3	4
Never	Rarely	Repeatedly	Regularly	Always

. . . I drank less than 2 l of fluids during the day.

0	1	2	3	4
Never	Rarely	Repeatedly	Regularly	Always

. . . I had muscle tension or cramps.

0	1	2	3	4
Never	Rarely	Repeatedly	Regularly	Always

. . . I got together with friends.

0	1	2	3	4
Never	Rarely	Repeatedly	Regularly	Always

. . . I felt successful.

0	1	2	3	4
Never	Rarely	Repeatedly	Regularly	Always

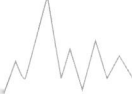

... I could barely unwind after work.

0	1	2	3	4
Never	Rarely	Repeatedly	Regularly	Always

... I had mood swings.

0	1	2	3	4
Never	Rarely	Repeatedly	Regularly	Always

... I was able to unwind after work.

0	1	2	3	4
Never	Rarely	Repeatedly	Regularly	Always

Score

Please keep in mind that this score only includes the past seven days and that there is a verifiable discrepancy between subjective impressions and scientific analysis.

Add up your points:

< 60 points = good energy status.

> 60 points = slight optimization requirement

> 70 points = definite optimization requirement

> 80 points = urgent optimization requirement

ENERGY SELF-CHECK FOR TOP COMPETITIVE ATHLETES

This self-check includes a series of findings regarding your mental and physical state and activities over the past two months.

In the last two months . . .

. . . I slept badly on days with intense training and competitions.

0	1	2	3	4
Never	Rarely	Repeatedly	Regularly	Always

. . . I had night sweats (unrelated to weather) and my clothing was damp when I woke in the morning.

0	1	2	3	4
Never	Rarely	Repeatedly	Regularly	Always

. . . I felt increasingly tired after intense training units.

0	1	2	3	4
Never	Rarely	Repeatedly	Regularly	Always

. . . I required longer regeneration phases.

0	1	2	3	4
Never	Rarely	Repeatedly	Regularly	Always

. . . I suffered from increasing mental fatigue.

0	1	2	3	4
Never	Rarely	Repeatedly	Regularly	Always

. . . I performed well in a competition/game.

0	1	2	3	4
Never	Rarely	Repeatedly	Regularly	Always

. . . I have experienced frequent performance fluctuations.

0	1	2	3	4
Never	Rarely	Repeatedly	Regularly	Always

. . . I harbored feelings of discord.

0	1	2	3	4
Never	Rarely	Repeatedly	Regularly	Always

. . . I did not feel completely physically fit.

0	1	2	3	4
Never	Rarely	Repeatedly	Regularly	Always

. . . I felt faint.

0	1	2	3	4
Never	Rarely	Repeatedly	Regularly	Always

. . . I had illnesses that prevented me from training regularly.

0	1	2	3	4
Never	Rarely	Repeatedly	Regularly	Always

. . . I was in a good mood.

0	1	2	3	4
Never	Rarely	Repeatedly	Regularly	Always

. . . I was dissatisfied with myself.

0	1	2	3	4
Never	Rarely	Repeatedly	Regularly	Always

. . . I was very indignant when criticized.

0	1	2	3	4
Never	Rarely	Repeatedly	Regularly	Always

. . . I had trouble getting motivated in the morning.

0	1	2	3	4
Never	Rarely	Repeatedly	Regularly	Always

. . . I did not feel very sprightly and dynamic.

0	1	2	3	4
Never	Rarely	Repeatedly	Regularly	Always

. . . I felt energized.

0	1	2	3	4
Never	Rarely	Repeatedly	Regularly	Always

. . . I suffered from increasing overload reactions of the tendon-ligament apparatus.

0	1	2	3	4
Never	Rarely	Repeatedly	Regularly	Always

. . . I preferred white pasta and rice on training days.

0	1	2	3	4
Never	Rarely	Repeatedly	Regularly	Always

. . . I drank mineral water containing > 1,500 mg/l of hydrogen carbonate.

0	1	2	3	4
Never	Rarely	Repeatedly	Regularly	Always

. . . I was able to fully tap my performance potential.

0	1	2	3	4
Never	Rarely	Repeatedly	Regularly	Always

. . . I had minor injuries.

0	1	2	3	4
Never	Rarely	Repeatedly	Regularly	Always

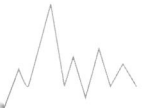

. . . I ate 600-800 g of fruit and vegetables every day.

0	1	2	3	4
Never	Rarely	Repeatedly	Regularly	Always

. . . I had the right attitudes during competitions.

0	1	2	3	4
Never	Rarely	Repeatedly	Regularly	Always

. . . I was convinced that I reached my training goals.

0	1	2	3	4
Never	Rarely	Repeatedly	Regularly	Always

. . . I felt completely overwhelmed.

0	1	2	3	4
Never	Rarely	Repeatedly	Regularly	Always

. . . I was able to focus well during training and competitions.

0	1	2	3	4
Never	Rarely	Repeatedly	Regularly	Always

. . . I was physically exhausted and fell asleep in front of the TV.

0	1	2	3	4
Never	Rarely	Repeatedly	Regularly	Always

. . . I lacked mental crispness.

0	1	2	3	4
Never	Rarely	Repeatedly	Regularly	Always

. . . I reacted with irritation in my personal sphere.

0	1	2	3	4
Never	Rarely	Repeatedly	Regularly	Always

Score

Please keep in mind that this score only includes the past two months and that there is a verifiable discrepancy between subjective impressions and scientific analysis.

Add up your points:

< 50 points = good energy status.

> 50 points = slight optimization requirement

> 60 points = definite optimization requirement

> 70 points = urgent optimization requirement

6   PHOTO CREDITS

Cover design:	Sabine Groten
Cover photo:	©Stockbyte/Thinkstock
Composition:	www.satzstudio-hilger.de
Inside layout:	Claudia Sakyi
Inside photos:	©Stockbyte/Thinkstock (Chapter openers, pg. 11, 13, 74, 109, 146, 178, 201)
	©Wavebreak Media/Thinkstock (pg. 144)
	©Polka Dot/Thinkstock (pg. 173)
	©Digitial Vision/Thinkstock (pg. 223)
Illustrations:	www.satzstudio-hilger.de
Copyediting:	Elizabeth Evans

7   PDF DOWNLOAD

You can find the journal forms and self-tests in PDF format at:

Link: m-m-sports.com/extras/top-performance

Please use the following login and password codes:

ID: performance

PW: tKkHEWqxQq9m

APPENDIX

8 FOUNDATION FOR MICRONUTRIENTS - PREVENTION, HEALTH, QUALITY OF LIFE

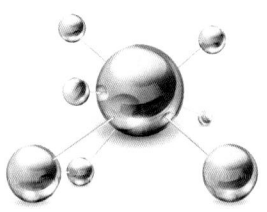

Foundation for Micronutrients – Prevention, Health, Quality of Life Non-profit LLC

The various overload reactions and associated disorders can verifiably be prevented with an optimal energy intake.

However, to date the scientific community denies these relationships.

According to statements made by international scientists, knowledge regarding the positive effects of a targeted micronutrient intake "is limited." It is still in the early stages of development.

His 15-plus years of positive experience and to date 38,000 compiled case reports have prompted Prof. Dr. Elmar Wienecke—sport scientist and founder of SALUTO The Competence Center for Health and Fitness—to establish the Foundation for Micronutrients, Prevention, Health, Quality of Life.

A team of physicians, sport scientists, biologists, natural scientists, and nutritionists conduct the research and practice-oriented application of new adjuvant and alternative capabilities in the area of micronutrient therapy.

FOUNDATION GOALS

Prevention

Establishing micronutrient therapy in a demographically-aging population with relation to age, sex, lifestyle, and prior illnesses.

Research

The early detection of biochemical disorders.

The practical application in the field of molecular biological micronutrient therapy in active people (recreational, competitive, elite sports).

The creation of discussion forums, significance of micronutrient intake in complementary medicine.

The advancement of science concerning microbiological micronutrient therapy by informing the public and providing basic knowledge on the true benefits of micronutrients. Integration of basic knowledge into the training structure of physicians, physical therapists, nutritionists.

PUBLICATIONS AND STUDIES

Creation of an endowment chair with various research tasks in the field of movement and micronutrient therapy.

Orthomolecular research will ensure the early detection of biochemical disorders so these may be counteracted with an optimal energy and micronutrient intake. In addition, the endowment chair shall be integrated as much as possible into different courses of study (Master of Mental and Physical Energy).

FOR YOU

If you are interested in supporting the Foundation for Micronutrient's concept and work, we would love to hear from you!

The foundation's pursuits are exclusively not-for-profit.

Foundation Chair: Prof. Dr. Elmar Wienecke

www.stiftung-mikronaehrstoffe.de

Email: stiftungmikronaehrstoffe@t-online.de

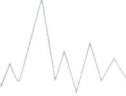 TOP PERFORMANCE IN BUSINESS AND SPORTS

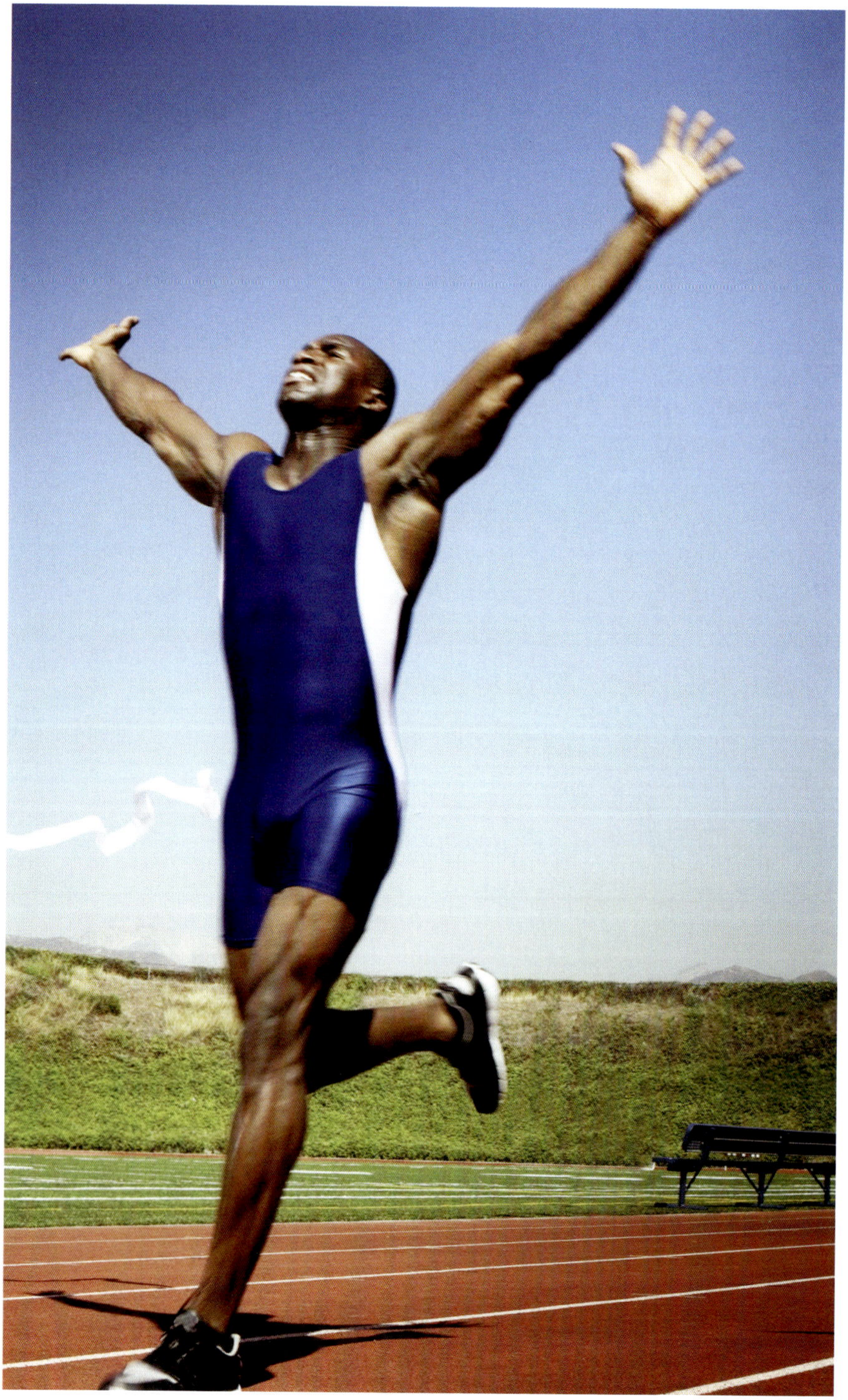

9 STATEMENTS

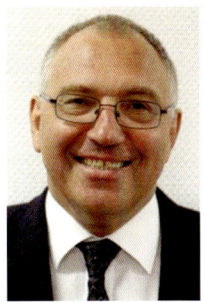

Peter Frese, president, DJB (German Judo Association)

"In recent years, our athletes have optimally benefitted from this concept. Prescription for Energy has verifiably allowed the athletes to optimally increase their performance capacity by being able to tap their full potential without injury. All of them feel considerably better mentally and physically, and in our sport that is of critical importance."

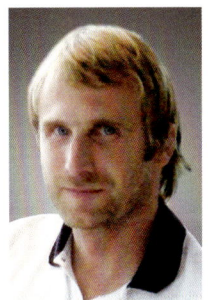

Daniel Bierofka (professional soccer player)

"After 17 surgeries that were mostly the result of repeated overload reactions, I have benefitted from Prescription for Energy for the past four years, 2008-2012, and was able to complete nearly every game for my team. I feel mentally and physically better than I have in a long time. I am certain that if my friend Horst Allmann had told me about this truly unique energy concept sooner I would have been able to avoid many injuries. The continuous, individualized formula showed me that I no longer have to tap into my body's own cartilage and bone metabolism reserves in order to achieve long-term optimal performance."

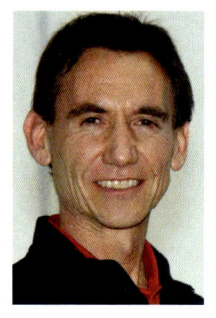

Dr. Kurt Mosetter (director, Center for Interdisciplinary Therapies [ZIT] in Constance, Germany, initiator of Myoreflex Therapy, team physician for the US national soccer team).

"The experience, the knowledge, and the highly individualized results behind Prof. Dr. Elmar Wienecke's energy metabolism and performance concept ensure a high degree of efficiency in all who use it. Better, faster, and more vital regeneration, performance optimization, and prevention blend seamlessly within this concept. I learned about SALUTO and Elmar Wienecke from my friend and training control expert Stefan Mücke. We were familiar with the basic aspects of energy metabolism such as the citric acid cycle. Therefore the developments in measuring individual way stations of the amino acid and energy metabolisms and providing optimum individual analyses are marvelous. All our clients, patients, and pro athletes enjoy the physical and neuromental benefits of SALUTO's performance optimizations."

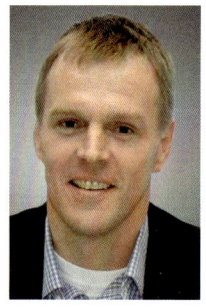

DHB (German Handball Federation) national team trainer **Martin Heuberger** (former trainer of the junior national team; world champions 2009, 2011)

"From 2006 to 2011, my junior national players were able to optimally benefit from this unique, integrated prevention concept. Next to your meticulous work with respect to performance diagnostics, the Prescription for Energy concept was an important puzzle piece in the performance development of my players."